BRAIN CANCER COOKBOOK FOR BEGINNERS

Nourishing Recipes with Expert Guidance for Strength, Healing, and Hope on Your Journey to Wellness

Kingsley Klopp

Table of Content

Vegetables

Fish and Seafood Recipes

Poultry Recipes

Soup & Stew Recipes

We're so glad you're here, taking proactive steps towards nourishing your body through this journey. Before you dive into the recipes, we want to share an important note.

Everyone's experience with brain cancer is unique, and so are their dietary needs. The recipes in this book are crafted with care and intention, focusing on ingredients that support general well-being and recovery. However, it's crucial to remember that what works for one person might not be ideal for another. Your body is your best guide, and your healthcare team is your best resource.

Please use these recipes as a foundation and feel free to adjust them to suit your individual needs and preferences. If you ever find yourself unsure about a particular ingredient or recipe, we strongly encourage you to consult with your doctor or a registered dietitian. They can provide personalized advice based on your specific health condition and treatment plan.

Additionally, we've included approximate nutritional information for each recipe. These values are estimates and can vary depending on the exact ingredients and brands you use. Cooking is as much about adaptation as it is about following instructions, so don't hesitate to make these dishes your own.

Furthermore, If our cookbook has brought joy to your kitchen and table, we'd be thrilled to hear about your experiences in an Amazon review. On the flip side, if you stumble upon any hiccups while exploring our recipes, don't hesitate to get in touch at **kloppkingsley@gmail.com.** We're here to support your cooking journey every step of the way

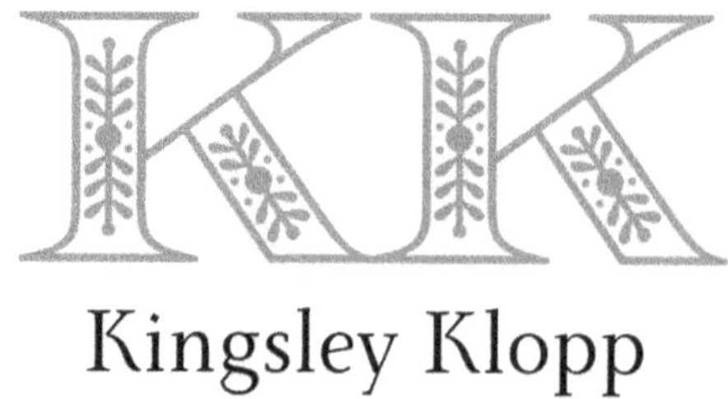

Kingsley Klopp

Introduction.

Hey there! If you've picked up this book, chances are you or someone you love is facing the tough journey of brain cancer. First off, let's acknowledge the elephant in the room: this is hard. No one ever expects to find themselves flipping through a cookbook specifically tailored for brain cancer patients, but here you are, and I'm so glad you are. You're already taking a brave step towards making this journey a bit easier, a bit healthier, and a lot more flavorful.

Now, let's talk about why this book exists. Nutrition plays a crucial role in supporting the body during cancer treatment. The right foods can boost your energy, help manage symptoms, and improve your overall well-being. But let's be real: figuring out what to eat can be overwhelming when you're dealing with everything else that comes with a cancer diagnosis. You're bombarded with medical jargon, treatment plans, and emotional ups and downs. The last thing you need is the added stress of planning meals. That's where this book comes in. We've compiled a collection of recipes that are not just nutritious but also easy to prepare and delicious to eat. We understand that your appetite might be unpredictable, and some days you might not feel like eating at all. These recipes are designed to be gentle on your stomach, packed with essential nutrients, and, most importantly, they taste good. Because even in the toughest times, food should be something you look forward to.

Think of this cookbook as your kitchen companion, here to guide you through the ups and downs of treatment. Whether you're craving a comforting bowl of soup, a hearty main dish, or a quick snack, we've got you covered. Each recipe is crafted with love and care, focusing on ingredients that support your health and recovery. We'll also sprinkle in some tips and tricks for making meal prep easier, because let's face it, no one wants to spend hours in the kitchen when they're not feeling their best. From batch cooking to freezer-friendly meals, we'll help you streamline your time in the kitchen so you can focus on what matters most: healing and spending time with loved ones.

So, take a deep breath and dive in. This journey might be challenging, but with the right nourishment, you can fuel your body and soul. Let's cook up some hope, one meal at a time.

Chapter 1: Understanding Brain Cancer

Types of Brain Cancer.

Brain cancer is a complex and challenging disease that arises from abnormal growths of cells in the brain. These abnormal growths, or tumors, can be benign (non-cancerous) or malignant (cancerous). Understanding the different types of brain cancer is crucial for diagnosis, treatment, and managing the disease. There are several types of brain cancer, each with distinct characteristics and implications.

Primary vs. Secondary Brain Cancer
Brain cancer is broadly categorized into primary and secondary (metastatic) brain cancers. Primary brain cancers originate in the brain, while secondary brain cancers start elsewhere in the body and spread to the brain.

Primary Brain Cancer
Primary brain cancers are less common but are significant due to their direct impact on brain function. They are further classified based on the type of cells they originate from and their location within the brain. The main types include:

1. **Gliomas**

Gliomas are the most common type of primary brain cancer, accounting for about 30% of all brain tumors and 80% of malignant brain tumors. They originate from glial cells, which support and protect neurons. Gliomas are classified into several subtypes based on the specific glial cell involved:

- Astrocytomas: These tumors arise from astrocytes, star-shaped glial cells. They range from low-grade (slow-growing) to high-grade (fast-growing and aggressive) tumors. The most severe form is glioblastoma multiforme, a highly malignant and aggressive cancer.
- Oligodendrogliomas: Originating from oligodendrocytes, these tumors are usually slower-growing and often occur in the cerebral hemispheres. They can be challenging to treat due to their tendency to infiltrate surrounding brain tissue.
- Ependymomas: These tumors develop from ependymal cells lining the ventricles of the brain and the central canal of the spinal cord. They can occur at any age but are more common in children and young adults.

2. **Meningiomas**
Meningiomas are typically benign tumors that develop from the meninges, the protective membranes covering the brain and spinal cord. They account for about 30% of primary brain tumors. While usually non-cancerous, their location can lead to significant neurological problems. Meningiomas are more common in women and tend to grow slowly, often discovered incidentally during imaging for other issues.

3. Medulloblastomas

These highly malignant tumors are most commonly found in children and originate in the cerebellum, the part of the brain responsible for coordination and balance. Medulloblastomas are fast-growing and can spread to other parts of the brain and spinal cord via cerebrospinal fluid. They require aggressive treatment, including surgery, radiation, and chemotherapy.

4. Schwannomas

Schwannomas, also known as acoustic neuromas, arise from Schwann cells that produce the myelin sheath covering nerves. These tumors are usually benign and develop on the nerves responsible for balance and hearing. While they grow slowly, their location can lead to hearing loss, balance issues, and facial nerve dysfunction.

5. Pituitary Adenomas

These tumors develop in the pituitary gland, a small gland at the base of the brain responsible for hormone production and regulation. Pituitary adenomas are generally benign but can affect hormone levels and cause various symptoms, depending on the hormones involved. They can be categorized as functioning (producing hormones) or non-functioning (not producing hormones).

6. Primary Central Nervous System Lymphomas

These rare tumors originate from lymphocytes, a type of white blood cell, within the brain or spinal cord. They are aggressive and often associated with immunocompromised individuals, such as those with HIV/AIDS or organ transplant recipients. Treatment typically involves a combination of chemotherapy and radiation.

Secondary (Metastatic) Brain Cancer

Secondary brain cancers are more common than primary brain cancers. They occur when cancer cells from other parts of the body spread to the brain. Common primary sites for cancers that metastasize to the brain include the lungs, breasts, kidneys, and skin (melanoma). These metastatic brain tumors are typically treated based on the origin of the primary cancer and may involve a combination of surgery, radiation, and systemic therapies like chemotherapy or targeted treatments.

Diagnosis and Treatment

Diagnosing brain cancer involves a combination of neurological exams, imaging studies (such as MRI and CT scans), and biopsy procedures to determine the tumor type and grade. Treatment strategies vary based on the type, location, and stage of the tumor, as well as the patient's overall health and preferences. Common treatments include:

- Surgery: The primary approach for accessible tumors, aiming to remove as much of the tumor as possible.
- Radiation Therapy: Uses high-energy beams to kill cancer cells or shrink tumors, often used post-surgery or for inoperable tumors.
- Chemotherapy: Involves drugs to kill cancer cells, typically used for malignant tumors and in combination with other treatments.

- Targeted Therapy: Uses drugs that specifically target cancer cell mechanisms, often with fewer side effects than traditional chemotherapy.
- Immunotherapy: Boosts the body's immune system to fight cancer cells, an emerging treatment option for certain brain cancers.

Symptoms and Diagnosis

Symptoms of Brain Cancer

Brain cancer symptoms can be diverse and are often related to the specific area of the brain affected by the tumor. Common symptoms include:

1. **Headaches**
   - Persistent or severe headaches, often worse in the morning or upon waking.
   - Headaches that change in pattern, intensity, or frequency.
   - Headaches accompanied by nausea or vomiting.
2. **Seizures**
   - New onset of seizures, especially in adults with no history of epilepsy.
   - Different types of seizures, including focal (affecting one part of the brain) and generalized (affecting the entire brain).
3. **Cognitive or Personality Changes**
   - Memory problems, confusion, or difficulty concentrating.
   - Changes in behavior, personality, or mood, such as increased irritability or depression.
4. **Motor and Sensory Deficits**
   - Weakness or numbness in one part of the body.
   - Difficulty with coordination or balance.
   - Problems with speech, vision, or hearing.
5. Nausea and Vomiting
   - Unexplained and persistent nausea or vomiting, often unrelated to other causes.
6. **Fatigue and Sleep Disturbances**
   - Persistent tiredness and a general sense of being unwell.
   - Difficulty sleeping or excessive sleepiness.
7. Other Symptoms
   - Difficulty swallowing or changes in the sense of taste or smell.
   - Hormonal imbalances, particularly with tumors affecting the pituitary gland.

Diagnosis of Brain Cancer

The diagnosis of brain cancer involves a series of steps, including a detailed medical history, neurological examination, and various diagnostic tests. Here's an overview of the diagnostic process:

1. **Medical History and Physical Examination**
   - Medical History: The physician will take a comprehensive medical history, noting any symptoms, their duration, and any family history of cancer or neurological disorders.
   - Neurological Examination: This includes testing reflexes, muscle strength, coordination, balance, sensation, and cranial nerve function.

2. Imaging Studies

- o Magnetic Resonance Imaging (MRI): The most commonly used imaging technique for diagnosing brain tumors. MRI provides detailed images of the brain and spinal cord, helping to identify the tumor's size, location, and potential spread.
- o Computed Tomography (CT) Scan: Useful for initial assessment, especially in emergencies. CT scans can quickly detect brain swelling, bleeding, and some types of tumors.
- o Positron Emission Tomography (PET) Scan: Often used to assess the metabolic activity of the tumor, helping to differentiate between benign and malignant tumors and to detect metastases.

3. Biopsy and Histopathological Examination

- o Stereotactic Biopsy: A minimally invasive procedure where a small sample of the tumor is removed using a needle guided by imaging technology. This sample is then analyzed under a microscope to determine the type and grade of the tumor.
- o Open Biopsy: Performed during surgery to remove the tumor. A portion of the tumor is sent to the lab for immediate analysis.

4. Lumbar Puncture (Spinal Tap)

- o This procedure involves collecting cerebrospinal fluid (CSF) to check for cancer cells or biomarkers indicating brain cancer, particularly useful in diagnosing certain types of tumors like medulloblastomas or lymphomas.

5. Advanced Diagnostic Tests

- o Molecular and Genetic Testing: Analyzes the tumor's genetic makeup to identify specific mutations or markers that can guide treatment decisions.
- o Electroencephalogram (EEG): Records electrical activity in the brain and can help identify seizure activity associated with brain tumors.

6. Functional MRI (fMRI) and Magnetoencephalography (MEG)

- o Functional MRI (fMRI): Measures brain activity by detecting changes in blood flow, useful for pre-surgical planning to avoid critical brain areas.
- o Magnetoencephalography (MEG): Maps brain function by recording magnetic fields produced by neuronal activity, aiding in precise tumor localization.

Combining Diagnostic Information

A multidisciplinary team of specialists, including neurologists, neurosurgeons, radiologists, and pathologists, reviews all diagnostic information to make an accurate diagnosis. The team considers the tumor's type, grade, location, and the patient's overall health to develop a comprehensive treatment plan.

Treatment Options

Surgical Treatment

Craniotomy

A craniotomy is the most common surgical procedure for brain tumors, involving the removal of a portion of the skull to access the brain. The surgeon aims to remove as much of the tumor as possible while minimizing damage to surrounding brain tissue. Types of craniotomies include:

- Awake Craniotomy: The patient is awake during surgery to help the surgeon avoid critical areas of the brain involved in speech and movement.
- Extended Craniotomy: Larger sections of the skull are removed to access deeper or more extensive tumors.

Stereotactic Surgery

This minimally invasive technique uses a 3D coordinate system to locate small brain tumors precisely. It allows for targeted biopsy, radiation, or surgery with minimal disruption to surrounding tissue.

Endoscopic Surgery

Endoscopic surgery involves using a small camera and surgical instruments inserted through a small incision or natural openings, such as the nostrils. This technique is particularly useful for tumors located in hard-to-reach areas like the pituitary gland.

Radiation Therapy

External Beam Radiation Therapy (EBRT)

EBRT is the most common form of radiation therapy for brain tumors. It involves directing high-energy beams at the tumor from outside the body. Techniques include:

- Three-Dimensional Conformal Radiation Therapy (3D-CRT): Uses 3D imaging to target the tumor precisely.
- Intensity-Modulated Radiation Therapy (IMRT): Modulates the intensity of the radiation beams to spare healthy tissue.
- Proton Beam Therapy: Uses protons instead of X-rays, delivering high doses of radiation to the tumor with minimal exposure to surrounding tissue.

Stereotactic Radiosurgery (SRS)

SRS delivers a high dose of radiation in a single session with extreme precision, using techniques like Gamma Knife or CyberKnife. It is suitable for small, well-defined tumors and inoperable cases.

Brachytherapy

This technique involves placing radioactive material directly inside or near the tumor. It provides high radiation doses to the tumor while sparing nearby healthy tissue. Brachytherapy is less commonly used for brain tumors but can be effective in specific cases.

Chemotherapy

Traditional Chemotherapy

Chemotherapy uses drugs to kill cancer cells or stop them from growing. Commonly used drugs for brain cancer include temozolomide (Temodar), often used in conjunction with radiation therapy. Chemotherapy can be administered orally, intravenously, or directly into the cerebrospinal fluid.

Targeted Therapy

Targeted therapy involves drugs that specifically target molecular pathways involved in tumor growth. These drugs tend to have fewer side effects than traditional chemotherapy. Examples include:

- Bevacizumab (Avastin): Targets the vascular endothelial growth factor (VEGF) pathway to inhibit the formation of new blood vessels that supply the tumor.
- Erlotinib (Tarceva): Inhibits the epidermal growth factor receptor (EGFR) pathway, which is often overactive in brain tumors.

Immunotherapy

Immunotherapy harnesses the body's immune system to fight cancer. Types of immunotherapy for brain cancer include:

Immune Checkpoint Inhibitors

These drugs block proteins that prevent the immune system from attacking cancer cells. Examples include nivolumab (Opdivo) and pembrolizumab (Keytruda).

Cancer Vaccines

Vaccines stimulate the immune system to recognize and attack cancer cells. For example, the DCVax vaccine is being studied for its potential to treat glioblastoma.

Adoptive Cell Transfer

This experimental therapy involves extracting immune cells from the patient, modifying them to better recognize cancer cells, and reinfusing them into the patient.

Experimental and Emerging Therapies

Tumor Treating Fields (TTF)

TTF uses alternating electric fields to disrupt cancer cell division. It is delivered through electrodes placed on the scalp and is used in conjunction with standard treatments for glioblastoma.

Gene Therapy

Gene therapy involves modifying the genetic material of cancer cells to stop their growth or make them more susceptible to other treatments. This approach is still largely experimental but holds promise for the future.

Supportive and Palliative Care
Symptom Management
Effective symptom management is crucial for maintaining the quality of life. This may include medications to control pain, seizures, nausea, and swelling.
Rehabilitation
Rehabilitation services, such as physical therapy, occupational therapy, and speech therapy, help patients regain lost function and adapt to changes caused by the tumor or treatment.
Psychological Support
Psychological support, including counseling and support groups, is essential for addressing the emotional and mental health needs of patients and their families.

Combination Therapies
Often, a combination of treatments is used to maximize efficacy and minimize side effects. For instance, surgery may be followed by radiation and chemotherapy. The choice of combination depends on various factors, including the type and grade of the tumor, its location, and the patient's overall health.

Personalized Treatment Plans
Advances in molecular biology and genomics have paved the way for personalized treatment plans tailored to the genetic profile of the tumor. This approach aims to improve outcomes by targeting specific characteristics of the tumor.

Hence, treating brain cancer is a complex process that requires a multidisciplinary approach and personalized treatment plans. The goal is to remove or reduce the tumor, manage symptoms, and improve the patient's quality of life. Advances in surgical techniques, radiation therapy, chemotherapy, and emerging treatments offer hope for better outcomes. Ongoing research and clinical trials continue to explore new and innovative ways to treat brain cancer and enhance the lives of those affected by this challenging disease.

Chapter 2: Essential Nutrients for Brain Cancer Patients

Proteins.

Protein is a vital nutrient for everyone, but it holds special significance for brain cancer patients. This macronutrient plays a crucial role in maintaining and repairing tissues, supporting the immune system, and preserving muscle mass, all of which are essential for individuals undergoing cancer treatment.

The Role of Protein in the Body

Proteins are made up of amino acids, which are the building blocks of the body's tissues and organs. They serve several critical functions, including:

- Tissue Repair and Growth: Protein is essential for repairing and building new tissues, particularly important for cancer patients who often experience tissue damage from treatments like surgery, radiation, and chemotherapy.
- Immune Function: Proteins are necessary for the production of antibodies and immune cells, which help the body fight infections and other diseases.
- Enzyme and Hormone Production: Many enzymes and hormones, which regulate various bodily functions, are proteins.
- Muscle Maintenance: Protein helps preserve muscle mass, which can be affected by cancer-related weight loss and treatment side effects.
- Energy Source: When carbohydrate and fat intake is insufficient, the body can use protein as an energy source.

Importance of Protein for Brain Cancer Patients

Brain cancer and its treatments can significantly impact the body's protein needs and utilization:

- Increased Metabolic Demand: Cancer and its treatment can increase the body's metabolic rate, leading to greater protein needs.
- Muscle Wasting (Cachexia): Many cancer patients experience cachexia, a condition characterized by severe muscle wasting and weight loss. Adequate protein intake is essential to help combat this condition.
- Immune System Support: Treatments like chemotherapy and radiation can weaken the immune system. Protein supports the production and function of immune cells, helping patients fend off infections.
- Healing and Recovery: Surgery and radiation can cause tissue damage that requires protein for repair and recovery.
- Side Effect Management: Protein can help manage side effects like fatigue, weakness, and poor wound healing, enhancing overall quality of life.

Recommended Protein Intake

The recommended protein intake for cancer patients varies based on individual factors such as weight, age, activity level, and the extent of the disease. General guidelines suggest:

- Adults: The average recommended dietary allowance (RDA) for protein is 46 grams per day for women and 56 grams per day for men. However, cancer patients often need more—ranging from 1.0 to 1.5 grams of protein per kilogram of body weight per day.
- Higher Needs: Some patients, particularly those undergoing intensive treatments or experiencing significant muscle wasting, may require even higher amounts, up to 2.0 grams per kilogram of body weight per day.

Sources of Protein

It is important to include a variety of protein sources in the diet to ensure a balanced intake of all essential amino acids. Protein sources can be categorized into animal-based and plant-based:

Animal-Based Sources:

- Lean Meats: Chicken, turkey, and lean cuts of beef and pork.
- Fish and Seafood: Salmon, tuna, cod, shrimp, and other seafood.
- Dairy Products: Milk, yogurt, cheese, and cottage cheese.
- Eggs: Whole eggs and egg whites.
- Poultry: Chicken and turkey, especially skinless to reduce fat intake.

Plant-Based Sources:

- Legumes: Beans, lentils, chickpeas, and peas.
- Nuts and Seeds: Almonds, walnuts, chia seeds, flaxseeds, and sunflower seeds.
- Whole Grains: Quinoa, brown rice, and whole wheat products.
- Soy Products: Tofu, tempeh, and edamame.
- Vegetables: Certain vegetables like spinach, broccoli, and Brussels sprouts contain modest amounts of protein.

Strategies to Ensure Adequate Protein Intake

Ensuring adequate protein intake can be challenging for brain cancer patients due to factors like reduced appetite, taste changes, nausea, and difficulty swallowing. Here are some strategies to help:

1. Small, Frequent Meals: Eating smaller, more frequent meals can help manage appetite loss and ensure a steady intake of protein throughout the day.
2. High-Protein Snacks: Incorporate high-protein snacks such as Greek yogurt, protein bars, nuts, and cheese.
3. Protein Supplements: Protein powders and shakes can be an effective way to boost protein intake, especially for those with difficulty eating solid foods.

4. Incorporate Protein-Rich Foods into Meals: Add beans or lentils to soups and salads, sprinkle nuts or seeds on cereals and yogurt, and include lean meats or tofu in stir-fries and casseroles.

5. Flavor Enhancers: Use herbs, spices, and marinades to improve the taste of foods, making them more appealing to those experiencing taste changes.

6. Texture Modifications: For patients with difficulty swallowing, modify food textures by pureeing or blending foods to make them easier to consume.

Monitoring and Adjusting Protein Intake

Regular monitoring of nutritional status is crucial for brain cancer patients. This involves:

- Nutritional Assessments: Regular assessments by healthcare professionals, including dietitians, to monitor weight, muscle mass, and overall nutritional intake.
- Blood Tests: Checking blood protein levels and other markers of nutritional status.
- Personalized Nutrition Plans: Adjusting dietary plans based on the patient's evolving needs and treatment responses.

In summary, protein is a critical nutrient for brain cancer patients, supporting tissue repair, immune function, muscle maintenance, and overall recovery. Ensuring adequate protein intake through a balanced diet, incorporating both animal and plant-based sources, and employing strategies to overcome eating challenges can significantly improve the health and quality of life for those battling brain cancer. Regular monitoring and personalized nutritional care are essential components of effective cancer treatment and recovery.

Carbohydrates

Carbohydrates are a crucial macronutrient for everyone, providing the primary source of energy for the body, particularly for the brain. For brain cancer patients, managing carbohydrate intake is especially important due to their unique metabolic needs and the side effects of cancer and its treatments.

The Role of Carbohydrates in the Body

Carbohydrates are broken down into glucose, which is the main fuel for the brain and muscles. They perform several essential functions, including:

- Energy Production: Carbohydrates are the body's preferred energy source, supplying the energy needed for daily activities and bodily functions.
- Brain Function: Glucose is the primary energy source for the brain, supporting cognitive functions, concentration, and mood.
- Sparing Protein: Adequate carbohydrate intake spares protein from being used for energy, allowing it to perform its primary roles in tissue repair and immune function.
- Preventing Ketosis: Sufficient carbohydrate intake prevents the body from entering ketosis, a state in which fat is used as the primary energy source, producing ketones that can affect metabolism.

Types of Carbohydrates

Carbohydrates are classified into two main types: simple carbohydrates and complex carbohydrates.

Simple Carbohydrates:

- Monosaccharides and Disaccharides: These are sugars composed of one or two sugar molecules, including glucose, fructose, sucrose, and lactose. They are quickly digested and absorbed, providing rapid energy.
- Sources: Fruits, honey, table sugar, and dairy products.

Complex Carbohydrates:

- Polysaccharides: These are long chains of sugar molecules, including starches and fibers. They take longer to digest, providing sustained energy and helping regulate blood sugar levels.
- Sources: Whole grains, legumes, vegetables, and starchy foods like potatoes and corn.

Importance of Carbohydrates for Brain Cancer Patients

Carbohydrates are particularly important for brain cancer patients due to their role in supporting energy levels, brain function, and overall health:

- Energy Provision: Cancer and its treatments can significantly increase the body's energy requirements. Carbohydrates provide a readily available energy source to meet these increased needs.

- Brain Health: The brain relies heavily on glucose for energy. Adequate carbohydrate intake helps maintain cognitive functions, mood stability, and overall neurological health.
- Digestive Health: Complex carbohydrates, particularly those high in fiber, promote digestive health, prevent constipation, and support a healthy gut microbiome, which can be compromised during cancer treatments.
- Managing Treatment Side Effects: Treatments such as chemotherapy and radiation can cause nausea, fatigue, and loss of appetite. Carbohydrates, especially in easily digestible forms, can help manage these symptoms and ensure sufficient energy intake.

Recommended Carbohydrate Intake

The recommended carbohydrate intake for brain cancer patients varies based on individual factors such as age, weight, activity level, and specific treatment protocols. General guidelines suggest:

- Total Carbohydrate Intake: Carbohydrates should make up about 45-65% of total daily caloric intake, as recommended for the general population. However, individual needs may vary.
- Focus on Complex Carbohydrates: Emphasizing complex carbohydrates over simple sugars can help maintain stable blood sugar levels and provide sustained energy.

Sources of Carbohydrates

Incorporating a variety of carbohydrate sources ensures a balanced intake of nutrients, including vitamins, minerals, and fiber. Key sources include:

Whole Grains:

- Examples: Brown rice, quinoa, whole wheat bread, oatmeal, and barley.
- Benefits: Provide sustained energy, essential nutrients, and fiber for digestive health.

Fruits and Vegetables:

- Examples: Apples, berries, oranges, leafy greens, carrots, and sweet potatoes.
- Benefits: Rich in vitamins, minerals, antioxidants, and fiber, supporting overall health and immune function.

Legumes:

- Examples: Beans, lentils, chickpeas, and peas.
- Benefits: High in protein, fiber, and complex carbohydrates, supporting sustained energy and digestive health.

Dairy and Dairy Alternatives:

- Examples: Milk, yogurt, cheese, and fortified plant-based milks.
- Benefits: Provide simple carbohydrates (lactose), protein, and essential nutrients like calcium and vitamin D.

Nuts and Seeds:
- Examples: Almonds, chia seeds, flaxseeds, and sunflower seeds.
- Benefits: Contain carbohydrates, healthy fats, protein, and fiber, contributing to balanced energy and nutrient intake.

Fats

Fats are a crucial component of a balanced diet and play a vital role in the health and well-being of brain cancer patients. They provide a concentrated source of energy, support cell structure, and help absorb fat-soluble vitamins. For brain cancer patients, managing fat intake is essential due to the increased metabolic demands of the body, the need for optimal nutrition during treatment, and the role of certain fats in brain health.

The Role of Fats in the Body

Fats perform several essential functions in the body, including:
- Energy Source: Fats provide a dense source of energy, with nine calories per gram, which is more than double the energy provided by carbohydrates and proteins.
- Cell Structure and Function: Fats are a key component of cell membranes, providing structure and facilitating the function of cells.
- Absorption of Vitamins: Fats aid in the absorption of fat-soluble vitamins (A, D, E, and K), which are crucial for various bodily functions.
- Hormone Production: Fats are involved in the synthesis of hormones that regulate numerous physiological processes.
- Brain Health: Certain fats, particularly omega-3 fatty acids, are critical for brain development, function, and maintaining cognitive health.

Importance of Fats for Brain Cancer Patients

For brain cancer patients, fats are particularly important due to their role in providing energy, supporting the immune system, and maintaining overall health:
- Increased Energy Needs: Cancer and its treatments can elevate the body's energy requirements. Fats provide a concentrated energy source that helps meet these increased demands.
- Weight Maintenance: Maintaining a healthy weight is crucial for brain cancer patients, as weight loss and muscle wasting (cachexia) are common issues. Adequate fat intake can help prevent these problems.
- Immune Function: Fats play a role in immune function by supporting the structure and function of immune cells.
- Cognitive Support: Omega-3 fatty acids, found in certain fish and plant oils, support brain health and may help manage symptoms related to brain function and cognition.

Types of Fats

Fats are categorized into several types based on their chemical structure and health effects:

Saturated Fats:

- Sources: Found in animal products like meat, butter, cheese, and certain plant oils such as coconut oil and palm oil.
- Health Impact: Excessive intake of saturated fats can raise cholesterol levels and increase the risk of cardiovascular disease. However, moderate consumption is necessary for overall health.

Unsaturated Fats:

- **Monounsaturated Fats:**
  - Sources: Olive oil, avocados, nuts, and seeds.
  - Health Impact: These fats help reduce bad cholesterol levels (LDL) and are beneficial for heart health.
- **Polyunsaturated Fats:**
  - Sources: Fatty fish (salmon, mackerel, sardines), flaxseeds, walnuts, and sunflower oil.
  - Health Impact: Includes essential fatty acids like omega-3 and omega-6, which support brain function, reduce inflammation, and promote heart health.

Trans Fats:

- Sources: Found in partially hydrogenated oils used in some processed and fried foods.
- Health Impact: Trans fats are harmful and should be avoided as they increase bad cholesterol (LDL) and decrease good cholesterol (HDL), raising the risk of heart disease.

Omega-3 Fatty Acids:

- Sources: Fatty fish, flaxseeds, chia seeds, and walnuts.
- Health Impact: Omega-3 fatty acids are particularly beneficial for brain health, reducing inflammation, and supporting overall cognitive function.

Recommended Fat Intake

The recommended fat intake for brain cancer patients should be balanced, providing sufficient energy and supporting overall health while avoiding excessive intake of harmful fats. General guidelines suggest:

- Total Fat Intake: Fat should make up about 20-35% of total daily caloric intake.
- Emphasis on Healthy Fats: Focus on consuming more unsaturated fats (both monounsaturated and polyunsaturated) while limiting saturated and trans fats.

Sources of Healthy Fats

Incorporating a variety of healthy fat sources ensures a balanced intake of essential fatty acids and other nutrients. Key sources include:

Olive Oil:
- Benefits: Rich in monounsaturated fats and antioxidants, olive oil supports heart health and reduces inflammation.
- Usage: Ideal for cooking, salad dressings, and drizzling over vegetables.

Avocados:
- Benefits: High in monounsaturated fats, fiber, and various vitamins and minerals.
- Usage: Can be added to salads, smoothies, or used as a spread.

Nuts and Seeds:
- Benefits: Provide a mix of healthy fats, protein, and fiber.
- Usage: Great as snacks, in salads, or added to cereals and yogurt.

Fatty Fish:
- Benefits: Rich in omega-3 fatty acids, which support brain health and reduce inflammation.
- Usage: Include fish like salmon, mackerel, and sardines in the diet several times a week.

Flaxseeds and Chia Seeds:
- Benefits: Excellent sources of omega-3 fatty acids, fiber, and antioxidants.
- Usage: Can be added to smoothies, cereals, or baked goods.

Plant Oils:
- Benefits: Oils like sunflower, safflower, and canola oil provide polyunsaturated fats.
- Usage: Suitable for cooking, baking, and salad dressings.

Strategies to Ensure Adequate Fat Intake

Ensuring adequate fat intake can be challenging for brain cancer patients due to symptoms like nausea, taste changes, and reduced appetite. Here are some strategies to help:

1. Incorporate Healthy Fats into Meals: Add avocados, nuts, seeds, and olive oil to salads, soups, and main dishes.
2. Choose Fatty Fish: Include fish like salmon and mackerel in meals, aiming for at least two servings per week.
3. Snack on Nuts and Seeds: Keep nuts and seeds handy for quick, healthy snacks.
4. Use Plant Oils: Cook with healthy oils like olive oil and canola oil instead of butter or margarine.
5. Add Fats to Smoothies: Blend in ingredients like nut butters, flaxseed oil, or avocado for a nutrient-rich smoothie.

Vitamins and Minerals

Vitamins and minerals are vital micronutrients required for numerous physiological functions, including immune response, energy production, and cellular repair. For brain cancer patients, ensuring adequate intake of these nutrients is crucial to support overall health, manage treatment side effects, and promote recovery.

The Role of Vitamins and Minerals

Vitamins and minerals perform a wide range of functions in the body:

- Immune Support: They enhance the body's ability to fight infections and illness.
- Energy Production: They are essential in the metabolic pathways that convert food into energy.
- Cellular Repair and Growth: They play a crucial role in the synthesis and repair of DNA and other cellular structures.
- Antioxidant Defense: Some vitamins and minerals act as antioxidants, protecting cells from damage caused by free radicals.

Important Vitamins for Brain Cancer Patients

Vitamin A:

- Benefits: Essential for immune function, vision, and cellular growth.
- Sources: Carrots, sweet potatoes, spinach, and dairy products.
- Role for Brain Cancer Patients: Supports immune health, which is critical during and after cancer treatment.

B Vitamins (B1, B2, B3, B6, B9, B12):

- Benefits: Crucial for energy production, brain function, and the formation of red blood cells.
- Sources: Whole grains, meats, eggs, dairy products, legumes, and leafy greens.
- Role for Brain Cancer Patients: Helps manage fatigue, supports cognitive function, and aids in the repair of DNA.

Vitamin C:

- Benefits: Supports the immune system, acts as an antioxidant, and promotes wound healing.
- Sources: Citrus fruits, strawberries, bell peppers, and broccoli.
- Role for Brain Cancer Patients: Enhances immune defense and aids in recovery post-surgery.

Vitamin D:
- Benefits: Essential for bone health, immune function, and reducing inflammation.
- Sources: Sunlight exposure, fatty fish, fortified dairy products, and supplements.
- Role for Brain Cancer Patients: Supports bone health, which can be compromised by steroid treatments, and enhances immune function.

Vitamin E:
- Benefits: Acts as an antioxidant, protecting cells from oxidative stress.
- Sources: Nuts, seeds, spinach, and vegetable oils.
- Role for Brain Cancer Patients: Helps protect cells from damage caused by treatments like radiation and chemotherapy.

Vitamin K:
- Benefits: Essential for blood clotting and bone health.
- Sources: Leafy green vegetables, broccoli, and Brussels sprouts.
- Role for Brain Cancer Patients: Important for patients undergoing surgery to ensure proper blood clotting.

Important Minerals for Brain Cancer Patients

Calcium:
- Benefits: Essential for bone health, muscle function, and nerve signaling.
- Sources: Dairy products, leafy greens, almonds, and fortified plant milks.
- Role for Brain Cancer Patients: Supports bone health, especially important for patients on steroids, which can weaken bones.

Iron:
- Benefits: Necessary for the production of hemoglobin, which carries oxygen in the blood.
- Sources: Red meat, poultry, fish, lentils, and spinach.
- Role for Brain Cancer Patients: Prevents anemia, a common issue in cancer patients, and supports overall energy levels.

Magnesium:
- Benefits: Involved in over 300 biochemical reactions in the body, including energy production and muscle function.
- Sources: Nuts, seeds, whole grains, and leafy greens.
- Role for Brain Cancer Patients: Helps manage fatigue and muscle cramps, common side effects of treatment.

Selenium:
- Benefits: Acts as an antioxidant and supports immune function.
- Sources: Brazil nuts, seafood, and whole grains.
- Role for Brain Cancer Patients: Enhances antioxidant defense and supports overall immune health.

Zinc:
- Benefits: Essential for immune function, wound healing, and DNA synthesis.
- Sources: Meat, shellfish, legumes, and seeds.
- Role for Brain Cancer Patients: Supports immune function and aids in recovery post-surgery.

Strategies to Ensure Adequate Vitamin and Mineral Intake

Ensuring adequate intake of vitamins and minerals can be challenging for brain cancer patients due to treatment side effects like nausea, reduced appetite, and taste changes. Here are some strategies to help:

1. Diverse Diet: Aim to include a variety of foods from all food groups to cover the spectrum of essential vitamins and minerals.
2. Small, Frequent Meals: Eating smaller, more frequent meals can help manage appetite loss and ensure consistent nutrient intake.
3. Fortified Foods: Choose fortified foods, such as cereals and plant-based milks, to boost intake of specific vitamins and minerals.
4. Smoothies and Juices: Incorporate fruits and vegetables into smoothies and juices, which can be easier to consume and digest.
5. Supplements: Consider supplements to address specific deficiencies, especially when dietary intake is insufficient. Consult with healthcare providers before starting any supplements.
6. Cooking Methods: Use cooking methods that preserve nutrient content, such as steaming, roasting, or sautéing, rather than boiling.
7. Flavor Enhancers: Use herbs, spices, and flavorings to make foods more palatable, especially if taste changes are an issue.

Hydration Needs

Hydration is a critical aspect of health and well-being for everyone, but it holds particular importance for brain cancer patients. Proper hydration is essential for maintaining bodily functions, supporting treatment efficacy, managing side effects, and improving overall quality of life.

The Importance of Hydration
Water is fundamental to numerous physiological processes, including:
- Cellular Function: Water is vital for cellular activities, including nutrient transport, waste removal, and energy production.
- Temperature Regulation: Adequate hydration helps regulate body temperature through sweating and respiration.
- Joint Lubrication: Water keeps joints lubricated, which is essential for mobility and comfort.
- Digestive Health: Water aids in digestion, nutrient absorption, and prevents constipation.
- Brain Function: Proper hydration supports cognitive function, mood regulation, and overall brain health.

Hydration Needs for Brain Cancer Patients
Brain cancer patients often have increased hydration needs due to various factors related to their condition and treatment:
- Increased Metabolic Demand: Cancer and its treatment can increase metabolic rates, leading to higher fluid requirements.
- Treatment Side Effects: Chemotherapy, radiation, and other treatments can cause side effects like vomiting, diarrhea, and fever, all of which increase fluid loss.
- Medication: Some medications used in cancer treatment, such as diuretics, can lead to increased urination and fluid loss.
- Nutritional Needs: Proper hydration is essential for the digestion and absorption of nutrients, which is crucial for patients with compromised nutritional status.

Factors Influencing Hydration Needs
Several factors can influence the hydration needs of brain cancer patients:
- Age and Weight: Younger patients and those with higher body weights generally require more fluids.
- Activity Level: Physical activity increases fluid loss through sweat and respiration, necessitating higher fluid intake.
- Environmental Conditions: Hot and humid environments increase sweat production and fluid loss.
- Health Status: Coexisting health conditions, such as kidney disease or diabetes, can affect fluid balance and hydration needs.

Signs of Dehydration

Recognizing the signs of dehydration is crucial for timely intervention. Common signs and symptoms of dehydration include:

- Thirst: One of the earliest indicators of dehydration.
- Dry Mouth and Skin: Lack of moisture in the mouth and skin can signal dehydration.
- Dark Urine: Concentrated, dark-colored urine often indicates inadequate fluid intake.
- Fatigue: Dehydration can cause feelings of tiredness and low energy.
- Dizziness and Confusion: Severe dehydration can lead to dizziness, confusion, and even fainting.
- Decreased Urine Output: Producing little or no urine is a clear sign of dehydration.
- Headaches: Dehydration can cause or worsen headaches, particularly in brain cancer patients.

Strategies to Maintain Adequate Hydration

Maintaining adequate hydration requires a proactive approach, especially for brain cancer patients who may face challenges such as nausea, vomiting, and difficulty swallowing. Here are some effective strategies:

1. Regular Fluid Intake: Encourage frequent sips of water throughout the day rather than waiting until feeling thirsty.
2. Fluid-Rich Foods: Incorporate foods with high water content, such as fruits (watermelon, oranges, and strawberries) and vegetables (cucumbers, lettuce, and tomatoes).
3. Variety of Beverages: Offer a variety of beverages to make drinking more appealing, including herbal teas, clear broths, and diluted fruit juices.
4. Oral Hydration Solutions: Use oral rehydration solutions or sports drinks to replenish electrolytes lost through vomiting or diarrhea.
5. Small, Frequent Sips: For patients experiencing nausea, small, frequent sips of water or ice chips can help maintain hydration without overwhelming the stomach.
6. Monitoring Fluid Intake: Keep track of daily fluid intake to ensure it meets the recommended levels, adjusting as needed based on treatment side effects and activity levels.
7. Hydration Reminders: Use alarms or reminders to encourage regular drinking, especially for patients who may forget due to cognitive issues.
8. Temperature Preferences: Offer fluids at different temperatures (cold, room temperature, warm) to find what is most comfortable and appealing to the patient.
9. Infused Water: Enhance the flavor of water by infusing it with fruits, herbs, or cucumber slices to make it more palatable.

Recommended Fluid Intake

The recommended fluid intake for brain cancer patients varies based on individual factors. However, general guidelines suggest:

- Men: About 3.7 liters (or 13 cups) of total water intake per day, from all beverages and foods.
- Women: About 2.7 liters (or 9 cups) of total water intake per day, from all beverages and foods.
- Adjustments: Increase intake during hot weather, periods of increased physical activity, or when experiencing side effects like vomiting or diarrhea.

Foods to Avoid

Foods High in Processed Sugars
Examples: Candy, soda, pastries, cookies, and other sweets.
Reasons to Avoid:
- Increased Inflammation: High sugar intake can promote inflammation, which can negatively impact the body's ability to fight cancer.
- Blood Sugar Spikes: Processed sugars cause rapid spikes and crashes in blood sugar levels, leading to fatigue and irritability.
- Weight Gain: Excessive sugar consumption can lead to weight gain, which may complicate treatment and recovery.

Healthier Alternatives:
- Opt for natural sweeteners like honey or maple syrup in moderation.
- Choose fruits such as berries, apples, and pears to satisfy sweet cravings.

Processed and Red Meats
Examples: Bacon, sausages, hot dogs, deli meats, and red meats like beef and pork.
Reasons to Avoid:
- Carcinogens: Processed meats contain preservatives like nitrates and nitrites, which have been linked to an increased risk of cancer.
- High Fat Content: Red and processed meats are high in saturated fats, which can contribute to heart disease and inflammation.
- Digestive Issues: These meats can be hard to digest and may cause gastrointestinal discomfort, especially for patients undergoing treatment.

Healthier Alternatives:
- Choose lean proteins like chicken, turkey, and fish.
- Include plant-based proteins such as beans, lentils, and tofu.

Fried and Greasy Foods
Examples: French fries, fried chicken, potato chips, and other deep-fried items.
Reasons to Avoid:
- High Fat Content: Fried foods are typically high in unhealthy fats that can lead to weight gain and cardiovascular issues.
- Digestive Problems: Greasy foods can cause nausea, indigestion, and other gastrointestinal problems, which are common side effects of cancer treatments.
- Low Nutritional Value: These foods often lack essential nutrients and can contribute to poor overall nutrition.

Healthier Alternatives:
- Opt for baked, grilled, or steamed foods instead of fried options.
- Snack on raw vegetables, air-popped popcorn, or whole grain crackers.

Highly Processed Foods

Examples: Packaged snacks, instant noodles, frozen meals, and other convenience foods.

Reasons to Avoid:

- Additives and Preservatives: These foods often contain additives, preservatives, and artificial ingredients that may be harmful.
- High Sodium Content: Many processed foods are high in sodium, which can lead to high blood pressure and fluid retention.
- Low Nutritional Quality: Highly processed foods typically lack essential vitamins, minerals, and fiber.

Healthier Alternatives:

- Prepare meals from scratch using fresh ingredients to control what goes into your food.
- Choose whole foods like fresh vegetables, fruits, whole grains, and lean proteins.

Dairy Products High in Fat

Examples: Whole milk, full-fat cheese, butter, and cream.

Reasons to Avoid:

- High Saturated Fat Content: Full-fat dairy products can contribute to increased cholesterol levels and inflammation.
- Lactose Intolerance: Some cancer patients may develop lactose intolerance, causing digestive discomfort.

Healthier Alternatives:

- Opt for low-fat or non-fat dairy options like skim milk or low-fat yogurt.
- Consider dairy alternatives such as almond milk, soy milk, or oat milk.

Alcohol

Examples: Beer, wine, spirits, and cocktails.

Reasons to Avoid:

- Interference with Treatment: Alcohol can interfere with the effectiveness of chemotherapy and other cancer treatments.
- Dehydration: Alcohol acts as a diuretic, leading to dehydration, which is particularly harmful for cancer patients.
- Increased Risk of Complications: Alcohol consumption can increase the risk of liver damage, weaken the immune system, and exacerbate treatment side effects.

Healthier Alternatives:

- Drink water, herbal teas, or natural fruit juices.
- Consider non-alcoholic beverages or mocktails for social occasions.

High-Sodium Foods

Examples: Canned soups, salted snacks, processed meats, and certain condiments.

Reasons to Avoid:

- Fluid Retention: High sodium intake can cause the body to retain fluid, leading to swelling and discomfort.
- Increased Blood Pressure: Excessive sodium can contribute to high blood pressure, increasing the risk of cardiovascular issues.
- Kidney Strain: High sodium can strain the kidneys, which may already be under stress from cancer treatments.

Healthier Alternatives:

- Use herbs and spices to flavor food instead of salt.
- Choose low-sodium or no-salt-added versions of canned and processed foods.

Caffeine

Examples: Coffee, tea, energy drinks, and certain sodas.

Reasons to Avoid:

- Dehydration: Caffeine is a diuretic and can contribute to dehydration, which is detrimental for brain cancer patients.
- Sleep Disturbances: Caffeine can interfere with sleep, which is crucial for recovery and overall health.
- Increased Anxiety: High caffeine intake can increase feelings of anxiety and jitteriness, which may be particularly challenging for patients dealing with cancer-related stress.

Healthier Alternatives:

- Opt for caffeine-free herbal teas or decaffeinated coffee.
- Drink water infused with fruits or herbs for a refreshing alternative.

Breakfast Recipes

1. Scrambled Eggs with Spinach

Ingredients:
- 4 large eggs
- 1 cup fresh spinach leaves, chopped
- 1/4 cup low-fat milk
- 1 tablespoon olive oil
- 1/4 teaspoon turmeric
- 1/4 teaspoon garlic powder
- 1/4 teaspoon onion powder
- 1/8 teaspoon black pepper
- 1/8 teaspoon paprika

Instructions:
1. In a medium bowl, whisk together the eggs and milk until well combined.
2. Heat olive oil in a non-stick skillet over medium heat.
3. Add spinach to the skillet and cook until wilted, about 2-3 minutes.
4. Pour the egg mixture over the spinach and let it sit for a few seconds until it begins to set around the edges.
5. Gently stir the eggs with a spatula, adding turmeric, garlic powder, onion powder, black pepper, and paprika.
6. Continue to cook, stirring frequently, until the eggs are fully cooked but still moist, about 3-4 minutes.
7. Serve immediately.

Nutrition Info per Serving:
- Calories: 200
- Protein: 15g
- Carbohydrates: 3g
- Fat: 15g
- Fiber: 1g
- Sugar: 1g

Number of Servings:
- **2 servings**

Cooking Time:
- **10 minutes**

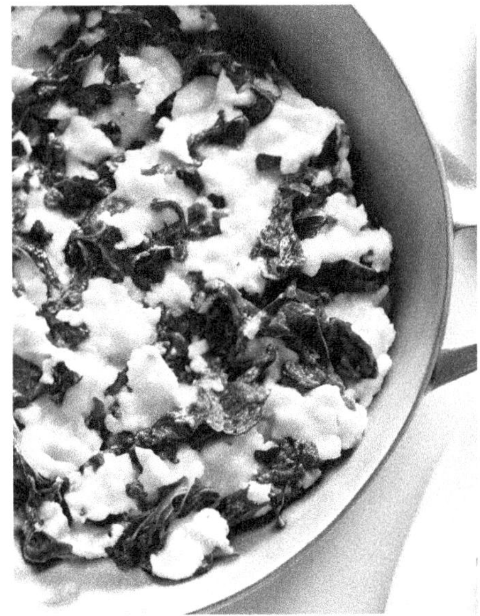

2. Banana Pancakes

Ingredients:

- 2 ripe bananas
- 2 large eggs
- 1/2 cup rolled oats
- 1/2 teaspoon baking powder
- 1/2 teaspoon vanilla extract
- 1/4 teaspoon cinnamon
- 1 tablespoon coconut oil (for cooking)
- Fresh berries and a drizzle of honey (optional, for serving)

Instructions:

1. In a blender, combine the bananas, eggs, rolled oats, baking powder, vanilla extract, and cinnamon. Blend until smooth.
2. Heat coconut oil in a non-stick skillet over medium heat.
3. Pour 1/4 cup of batter onto the skillet for each pancake. Cook until bubbles form on the surface and the edges look set, about 2-3 minutes.
4. Flip the pancakes and cook for an additional 1-2 minutes, until golden brown.
5. Serve with fresh berries and a drizzle of honey if desired.

Nutrition Info per Serving:

- Calories: 250
- Protein: 8g
- Carbohydrates: 40g
- Fat: 8g
- Fiber: 5g
- Sugar: 14g

Number of Servings:

- **2 servings (4 pancakes)**

Cooking Time:

- **15 minutes**

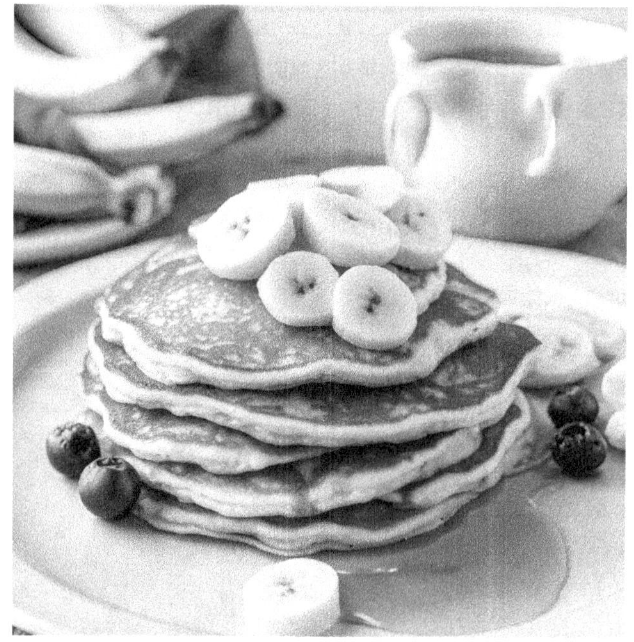

3. Smoothie Bowl

Ingredients:

- 1 ripe banana
- 1/2 cup frozen berries (blueberries, strawberries, or mixed berries)
- 1/2 cup unsweetened almond milk
- 1/4 cup plain Greek yogurt
- 1 tablespoon chia seeds
- 1 tablespoon honey
- Toppings: sliced banana, fresh berries, granola, and chia seeds

Instructions:

1. In a blender, combine the banana, frozen berries, almond milk, Greek yogurt, chia seeds, and honey. Blend until smooth and thick.
2. Pour the smoothie mixture into a bowl.
3. Top with sliced banana, fresh berries, granola, and a sprinkle of chia seeds.
4. Serve immediately.

Nutrition Info per Serving:

- Calories: 300
- Protein: 10g
- Carbohydrates: 55g
- Fat: 7g
- Fiber: 8g
- Sugar: 27g

Number of Servings:

- **1 serving**

Cooking Time:

- **10 minutes**

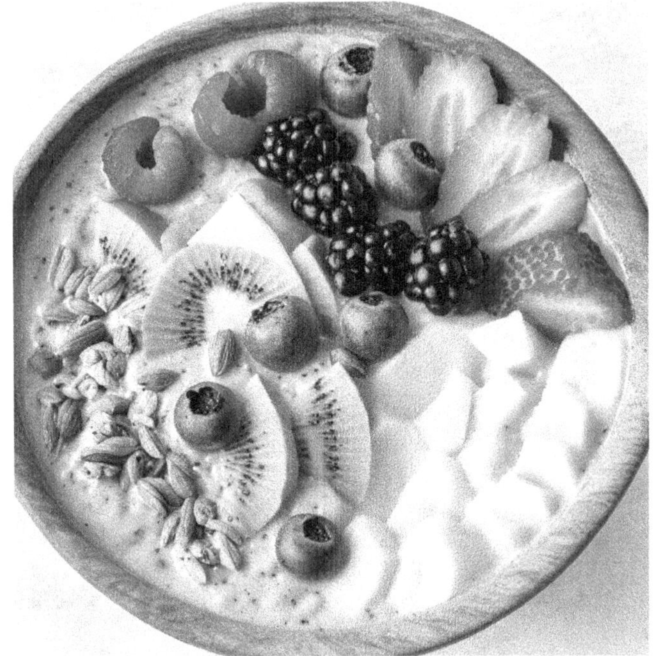

4. Oatmeal with Fresh Berries

Ingredients:

- 1 cup rolled oats
- 2 cups water
- 1/2 cup low-fat milk
- 1/2 teaspoon cinnamon
- 1 teaspoon vanilla extract
- 1 cup fresh berries (blueberries, raspberries, or strawberries)
- 1 tablespoon chia seeds
- 1 tablespoon honey or maple syrup

Instructions:

1. In a medium saucepan, bring water to a boil. Add rolled oats and reduce heat to a simmer.
2. Cook the oats, stirring occasionally, until the water is absorbed, about 5-7 minutes.
3. Stir in the milk, cinnamon, and vanilla extract. Continue to cook until the oats are creamy, about 2-3 more minutes.
4. Divide the oatmeal into bowls and top with fresh berries, chia seeds, and a drizzle of honey or maple syrup.
5. Serve immediately.

Nutrition Info per Serving:

- Calories: 250
- Protein: 7g
- Carbohydrates: 47g
- Fat: 6g
- Fiber: 8g
- Sugar: 14g

Number of Servings:

- 2 servings

Cooking Time:

- 15 minutes

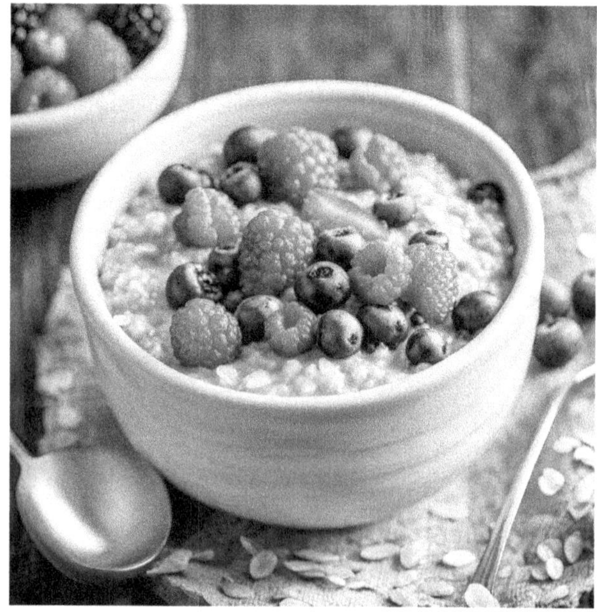

5. Apple Cinnamon Porridge

Ingredients:

- 1 cup rolled oats
- 2 cups water
- 1 cup low-fat milk
- 1 apple, peeled and diced
- 1/2 teaspoon ground cinnamon
- 1/4 teaspoon nutmeg
- 1 tablespoon chia seeds
- 1 tablespoon honey or maple syrup

Instructions:

1. In a medium saucepan, bring water to a boil. Add the rolled oats and reduce the heat to a simmer.
2. Cook the oats, stirring occasionally, for about 5-7 minutes, until the water is absorbed.
3. Stir in the milk, diced apple, cinnamon, and nutmeg. Continue to cook for another 5 minutes, until the apple is tender and the porridge is creamy.
4. Remove from heat and stir in the chia seeds and honey or maple syrup.
5. Serve immediately.

Nutrition Info per Serving:

- Calories: 300
- Protein: 8g
- Carbohydrates: 55g
- Fat: 6g
- Fiber: 8g
- Sugar: 18g

Number of Servings:

- **2 servings**

Cooking Time:

- **15 minutes**

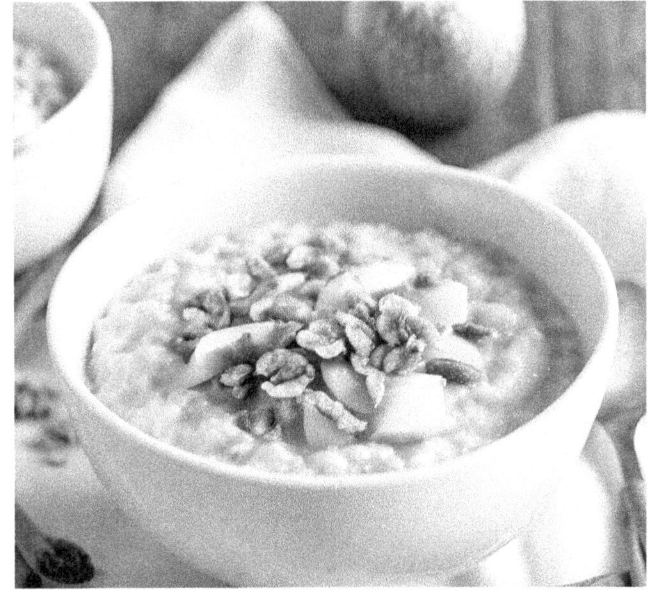

6. Egg and Vegetable Muffins

Ingredients:

- 6 large eggs
- 1/2 cup low-fat milk
- 1/2 cup chopped spinach
- 1/2 cup diced bell pepper
- 1/2 cup diced zucchini
- 1/4 cup diced onion
- 1/2 teaspoon garlic powder
- 1/2 teaspoon dried oregano
- 1/4 teaspoon paprika
- 1/4 teaspoon black pepper

Instructions:

1. Preheat the oven to 350°F (175°C) and grease a 12-cup muffin tin.
2. In a large bowl, whisk together the eggs and milk until well combined.
3. Stir in the chopped spinach, bell pepper, zucchini, onion, garlic powder, oregano, paprika, and black pepper.
4. Pour the egg mixture evenly into the muffin tin cups.
5. Bake for 20-25 minutes, until the muffins are set and slightly golden.
6. Allow the muffins to cool for a few minutes before removing them from the tin.
7. Serve immediately or store in the refrigerator for up to 3 days.

Nutrition Info per Serving:

- Calories: 100
- Protein: 8g
- Carbohydrates: 4g
- Fat: 6g
- Fiber: 1g
- Sugar: 2g

Number of Servings:

- **6 servings (2 muffins per serving)**

Cooking Time:

- **30 minutes**

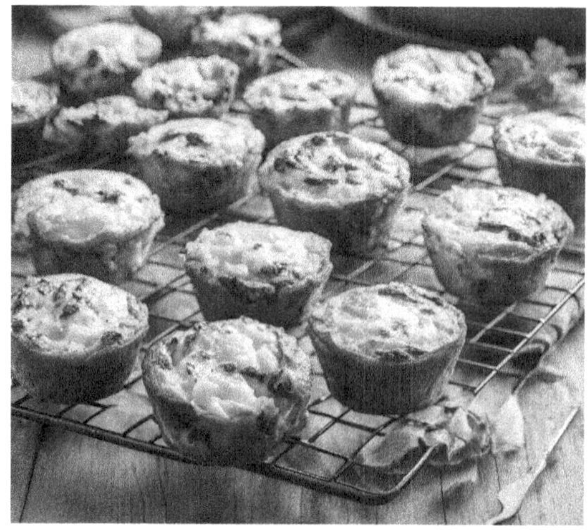

7. Sweet Potato Hash

Ingredients:

- 2 medium sweet potatoes, peeled and diced
- 1 tablespoon olive oil
- 1/2 cup diced red bell pepper
- 1/2 cup diced green bell pepper
- 1/4 cup diced onion
- 1/2 teaspoon garlic powder
- 1/2 teaspoon smoked paprika
- 1/4 teaspoon cumin
- 1/4 teaspoon black pepper
- 2 tablespoons chopped fresh parsley (optional, for garnish)

Instructions:

1. Heat the olive oil in a large skillet over medium heat.
2. Add the diced sweet potatoes to the skillet and cook for about 10 minutes, stirring occasionally, until they begin to soften.
3. Add the red bell pepper, green bell pepper, and onion to the skillet. Continue to cook for another 5-7 minutes, until the vegetables are tender and slightly caramelized.
4. Stir in the garlic powder, smoked paprika, cumin, and black pepper. Cook for an additional 2-3 minutes, until the spices are well incorporated.
5. Remove from heat and garnish with fresh parsley, if desired.
6. Serve immediately.

Nutrition Info per Serving:

- Calories: 150
- Protein: 2g
- Carbohydrates: 27g
- Fat: 5g
- Fiber: 5g
- Sugar: 8g

Number of Servings:

- **4 servings**

Cooking Time:

- **25 minutes**

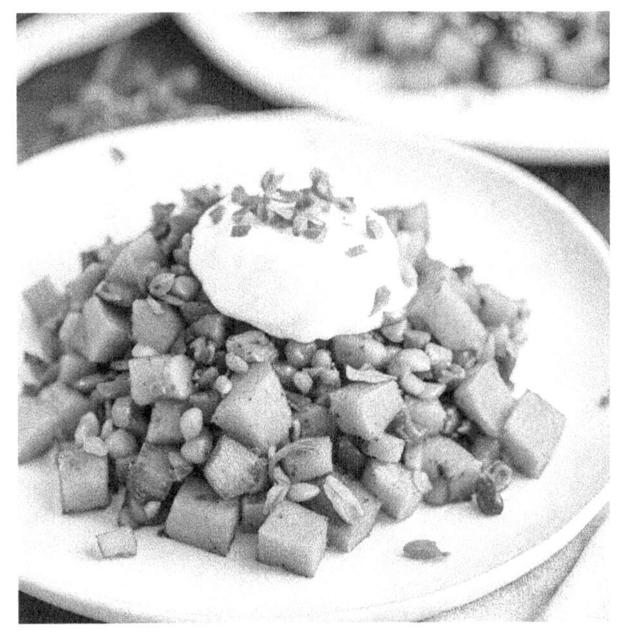

8. Quinoa and Berry Breakfast Bowl

Ingredients:

- 1 cup quinoa
- 2 cups water
- 1 cup mixed berries (blueberries, strawberries, raspberries)
- 1/2 cup low-fat Greek yogurt
- 1 tablespoon honey or maple syrup
- 1 tablespoon chia seeds
- 1/4 teaspoon ground cinnamon
- 1/4 teaspoon vanilla extract

Instructions:

1. Rinse the quinoa under cold water.
2. In a medium saucepan, bring the water to a boil. Add the quinoa, reduce heat to low, and cover. Simmer for 15 minutes or until the water is absorbed and the quinoa is tender.
3. Remove from heat and let it sit covered for 5 minutes, then fluff with a fork.
4. In a bowl, combine the cooked quinoa with Greek yogurt, honey or maple syrup, chia seeds, cinnamon, and vanilla extract.
5. Top with mixed berries.
6. Serve immediately.

Nutrition Info per Serving:

- Calories: 350
- Protein: 14g
- Carbohydrates: 65g
- Fat: 7g
- Fiber: 10g
- Sugar: 20g

Number of Servings:

- 2 servings

Cooking Time:

- 20 minutes

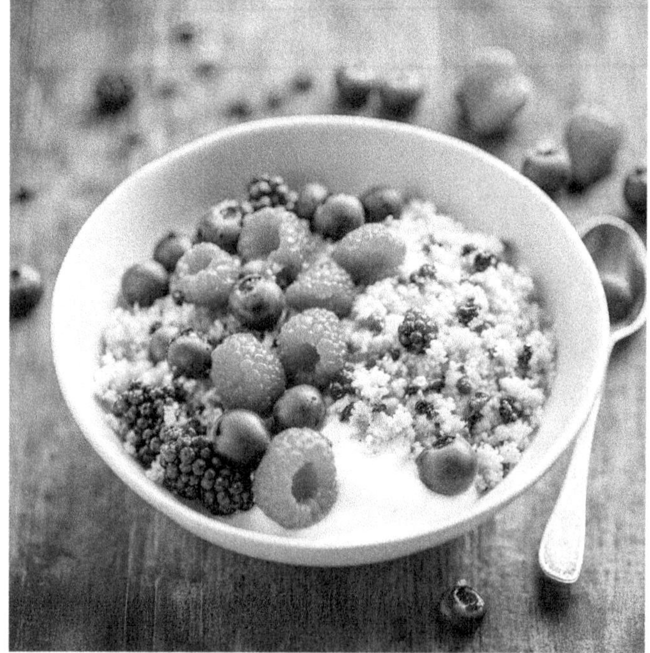

9. Turkey and Spinach Omelette

Ingredients:

- 4 large eggs
- 1/4 cup low-fat milk
- 1/2 cup cooked turkey breast, diced
- 1 cup fresh spinach, chopped
- 1/4 cup diced onion
- 1 tablespoon olive oil
- 1/4 teaspoon garlic powder
- 1/4 teaspoon paprika
- 1/4 teaspoon black pepper

Instructions:

1. In a medium bowl, whisk together the eggs and milk until well combined.
2. Heat olive oil in a non-stick skillet over medium heat.
3. Add the onion and cook until translucent, about 2-3 minutes.
4. Add the spinach and cook until wilted, about 2 minutes.
5. Add the cooked turkey breast and heat through, about 1-2 minutes.
6. Pour the egg mixture over the turkey and spinach. Let it cook without stirring until the edges start to set.
7. Gently lift the edges with a spatula, allowing the uncooked eggs to flow underneath. Continue until the omelette is mostly set, about 2-3 minutes.
8. Sprinkle garlic powder, paprika, and black pepper over the omelette.
9. Fold the omelette in half and cook for an additional minute.
10. Serve immediately.

Nutrition Info per Serving:

- Calories: 300
- Protein: 27g
- Carbohydrates: 5g
- Fat: 18g
- Fiber: 1g
- Sugar: 3g

Number of Servings:

- **2 servings**

Cooking Time:

- **15 minutes**

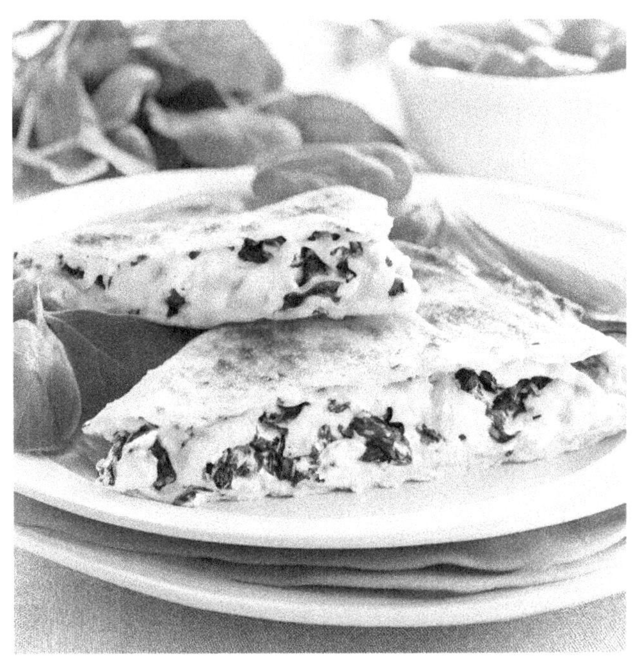

10. Almond Butter and Banana Sandwich

Ingredients:

- 4 slices whole grain bread
- 4 tablespoons almond butter
- 2 bananas, sliced
- 1 tablespoon honey (optional)

Instructions:

1. Toast the bread slices to your preference.
2. Spread 2 tablespoons of almond butter on each of two slices of bread.
3. Arrange the banana slices evenly over the almond butter.
4. Drizzle with honey if desired.
5. Top with the remaining slices of bread.
6. Serve immediately.

Nutrition Info per Serving:

- Calories: 350
- Protein: 9g
- Carbohydrates: 55g
- Fat: 14g
- Fiber: 7g
- Sugar: 20g

Number of Servings:

- **2 servings**

Cooking Time:

- **10 minutes**

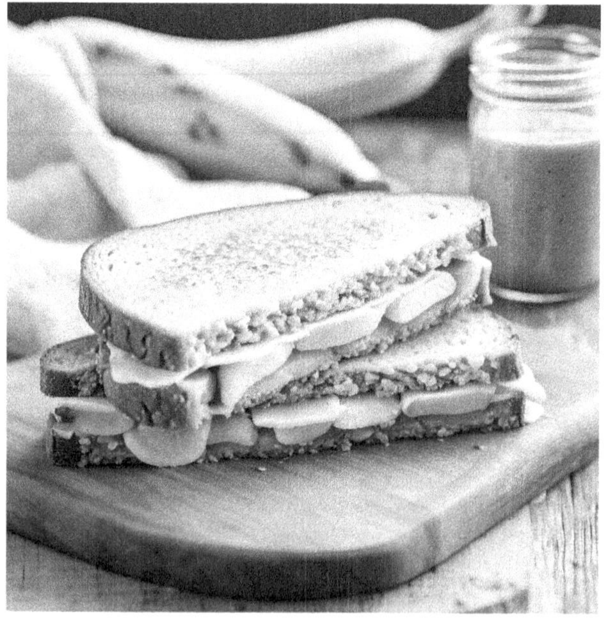

11. Chia Pudding

Ingredients:

- 1/4 cup chia seeds
- 1 cup unsweetened almond milk
- 1 tablespoon honey or maple syrup
- 1/2 teaspoon vanilla extract
- 1/2 cup mixed berries for topping

Instructions:

1. In a medium bowl, whisk together chia seeds, almond milk, honey or maple syrup, and vanilla extract.
2. Let the mixture sit for 5 minutes, then stir again to prevent clumping.
3. Cover the bowl and refrigerate for at least 4 hours, or overnight.
4. Before serving, stir the pudding and top with mixed berries.
5. Serve immediately.

Nutrition Info per Serving:

- Calories: 200
- Protein: 5g
- Carbohydrates: 25g
- Fat: 10g
- Fiber: 10g
- Sugar: 12g

Number of Servings:

- 2 servings

Cooking Time:

- **5 minutes prep time, plus 4 hours chilling**

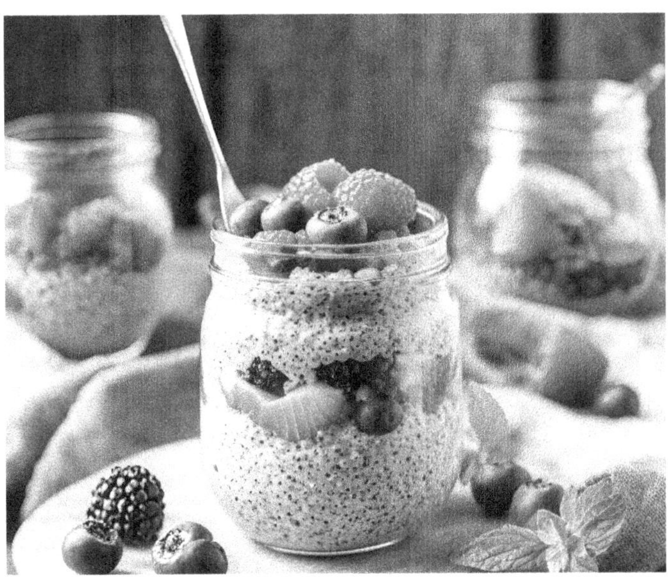

12. Buckwheat Pancakes

Ingredients:

- 1 cup buckwheat flour
- 1 tablespoon baking powder
- 1 tablespoon honey or maple syrup
- 1/2 teaspoon ground cinnamon
- 1 cup unsweetened almond milk
- 1 large egg
- 1 tablespoon coconut oil (for cooking)
- Fresh berries and a drizzle of honey (optional, for serving)

Instructions:

1. In a large bowl, whisk together the buckwheat flour, baking powder, and cinnamon.
2. In another bowl, combine the almond milk, egg, and honey or maple syrup. Whisk until well combined.
3. Pour the wet ingredients into the dry ingredients and stir until just combined.
4. Heat coconut oil in a non-stick skillet over medium heat.
5. Pour 1/4 cup of batter onto the skillet for each pancake. Cook until bubbles form on the surface and the edges look set, about 2-3 minutes.
6. Flip the pancakes and cook for an additional 1-2 minutes, until golden brown.
7. Serve with fresh berries and a drizzle of honey if desired.

Nutrition Info per Serving:

- Calories: 250
- Protein: 7g
- Carbohydrates: 40g
- Fat: 8g
- Fiber: 5g
- Sugar: 10g

Number of Servings:

- **4 servings (8 pancakes)**

Cooking Time:

- **20 minutes**

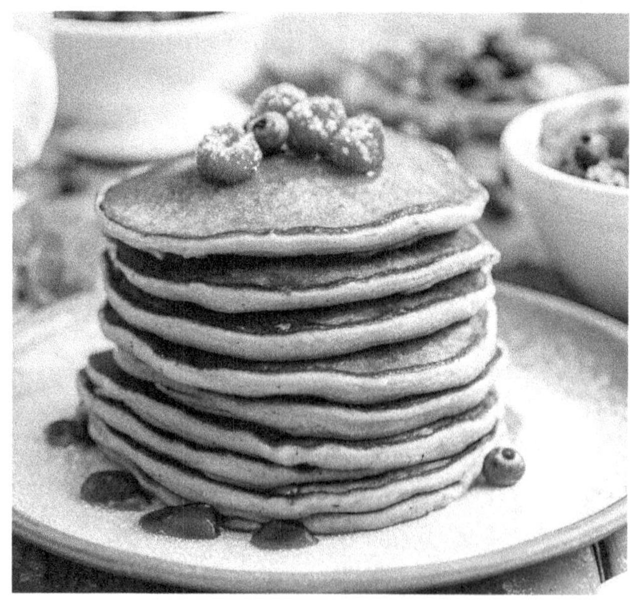

13. Kale and Mushroom Sauté

Ingredients:

- 2 tablespoons olive oil
- 1 cup mushrooms, sliced
- 2 cups kale, chopped
- 1/4 cup diced onion
- 2 cloves garlic, minced
- 1/4 teaspoon paprika
- 1/4 teaspoon thyme
- 1/8 teaspoon black pepper

Instructions:

1. Heat olive oil in a large skillet over medium heat.
2. Add the onions and cook until translucent, about 3 minutes.
3. Add the garlic and cook for another minute.
4. Add the mushrooms and cook until they release their juices and begin to brown, about 5 minutes.
5. Add the kale, paprika, thyme, and black pepper. Cook until the kale is wilted and tender, about 5 minutes.
6. Serve immediately.

Nutrition Info per Serving:

- Calories: 150
- Protein: 3g
- Carbohydrates: 10g
- Fat: 11g
- Fiber: 3g
- Sugar: 2g

Number of Servings:

- **2 servings**

Cooking Time:

- **15 minutes**

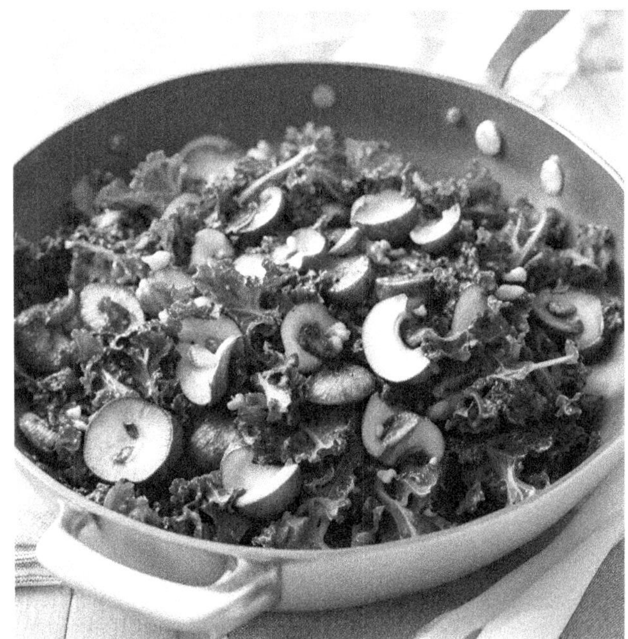

14. Baked Avocado Eggs

Ingredients:

- 2 ripe avocados
- 4 large eggs
- 1/4 teaspoon paprika
- 1/4 teaspoon garlic powder
- 1/4 teaspoon black pepper
- Fresh chives, chopped (optional, for garnish)

Instructions:

1. Preheat the oven to 425°F (220°C).
2. Cut the avocados in half and remove the pits. Scoop out a little of the flesh to make room for the eggs.
3. Place the avocado halves in a baking dish, making sure they are stable.
4. Crack an egg into each avocado half.
5. Sprinkle paprika, garlic powder, and black pepper over the eggs.
6. Bake for 15-20 minutes, or until the egg whites are set.
7. Garnish with fresh chives if desired.
8. Serve immediately.

Nutrition Info per Serving:

- Calories: 300
- Protein: 10g
- Carbohydrates: 12g
- Fat: 25g
- Fiber: 8g
- Sugar: 1g

Number of Servings:

- 2 servings

Cooking Time:

- 20 minutes

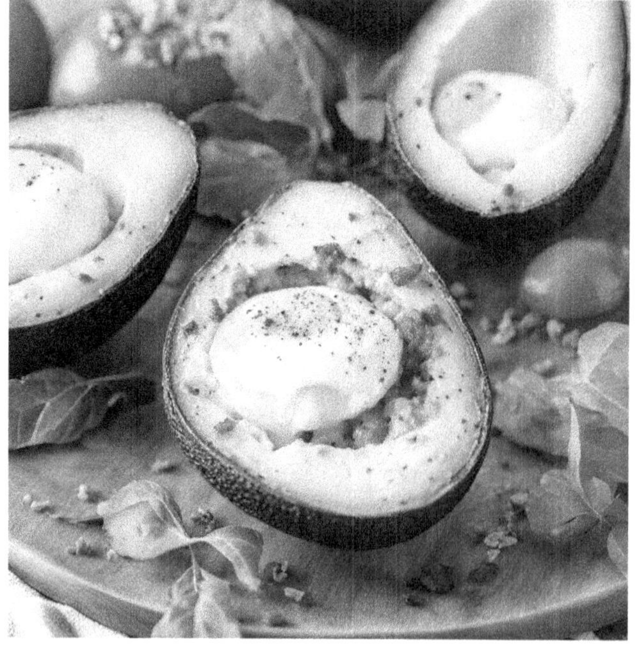

15. Millet Porridge

Ingredients:

- 1 cup millet
- 3 cups water
- 1 cup low-fat milk
- 1 tablespoon honey or maple syrup
- 1/2 teaspoon ground cinnamon
- 1/4 teaspoon nutmeg
- 1/4 cup chopped nuts (optional, for topping)
- Fresh fruit (optional, for topping)

Instructions:

1. Rinse the millet under cold water.
2. In a medium saucepan, bring water to a boil. Add the millet, reduce heat to low, and cover. Simmer for 20 minutes, or until the water is absorbed.
3. Stir in the milk, honey or maple syrup, cinnamon, and nutmeg. Cook for an additional 5-10 minutes, until the porridge is creamy.
4. Divide into bowls and top with chopped nuts and fresh fruit if desired.
5. Serve immediately.

Nutrition Info per Serving:

- Calories: 300
- Protein: 8g
- Carbohydrates: 55g
- Fat: 6g
- Fiber: 6g
- Sugar: 10g

Number of Servings:

- **4 servings**

Cooking Time:

- **30 minutes**

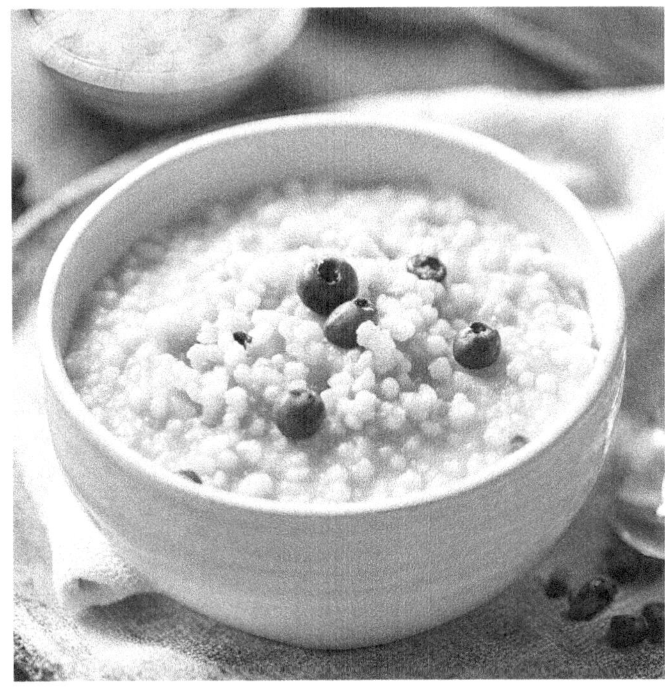

16. Zucchini Bread

Ingredients:

- 1 1/2 cups whole wheat flour
- 1 teaspoon baking soda
- 1/2 teaspoon baking powder
- 1 teaspoon ground cinnamon
- 1/2 teaspoon nutmeg
- 1/4 teaspoon black pepper
- 2 large eggs
- 1/2 cup applesauce
- 1/2 cup honey or maple syrup
- 1 teaspoon vanilla extract
- 1 1/2 cups grated zucchini
- 1/2 cup chopped walnuts (optional)

Instructions:

1. Preheat the oven to 350°F (175°C). Grease a 9x5 inch loaf pan.
2. In a large bowl, whisk together the whole wheat flour, baking soda, baking powder, cinnamon, nutmeg, and black pepper.
3. In another bowl, beat the eggs, applesauce, honey or maple syrup, and vanilla extract until well combined.
4. Add the wet ingredients to the dry ingredients and mix until just combined.
5. Fold in the grated zucchini and walnuts if using.
6. Pour the batter into the prepared loaf pan and smooth the top.
7. Bake for 50-60 minutes, or until a toothpick inserted into the center comes out clean.
8. Allow the bread to cool in the pan for 10 minutes, then transfer to a wire rack to cool completely.
9. Slice and serve.

Nutrition Info per Serving:

- Calories: 200
- Protein: 5g
- Carbohydrates: 35g
- Fat: 6g
- Fiber: 3g
- Sugar: 15g

Number of Servings:

- 10 servings

Cooking Time:

- 60 minutes

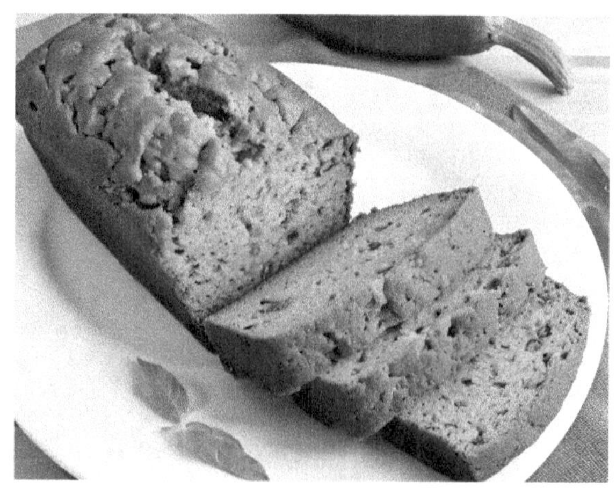

17. Tofu Scramble

Ingredients:

- 1 block firm tofu, drained and crumbled
- 1 tablespoon olive oil
- 1/2 cup diced bell pepper
- 1/2 cup diced onion
- 1 cup chopped spinach
- 1/4 teaspoon turmeric
- 1/4 teaspoon garlic powder
- 1/4 teaspoon cumin
- 1/4 teaspoon black pepper

Instructions:

1. Heat olive oil in a large skillet over medium heat.
2. Add the bell pepper and onion, and sauté until softened, about 5 minutes.
3. Add the crumbled tofu to the skillet and stir to combine.
4. Sprinkle with turmeric, garlic powder, cumin, and black pepper. Cook for about 5-7 minutes, stirring occasionally.
5. Add the spinach and cook until wilted, about 2-3 minutes.
6. Serve immediately.

Nutrition Info per Serving:

- Calories: 200
- Protein: 14g
- Carbohydrates: 10g
- Fat: 12g
- Fiber: 3g
- Sugar: 3g

Number of Servings:

- **2 servings**

Cooking Time:

- **15 minutes**

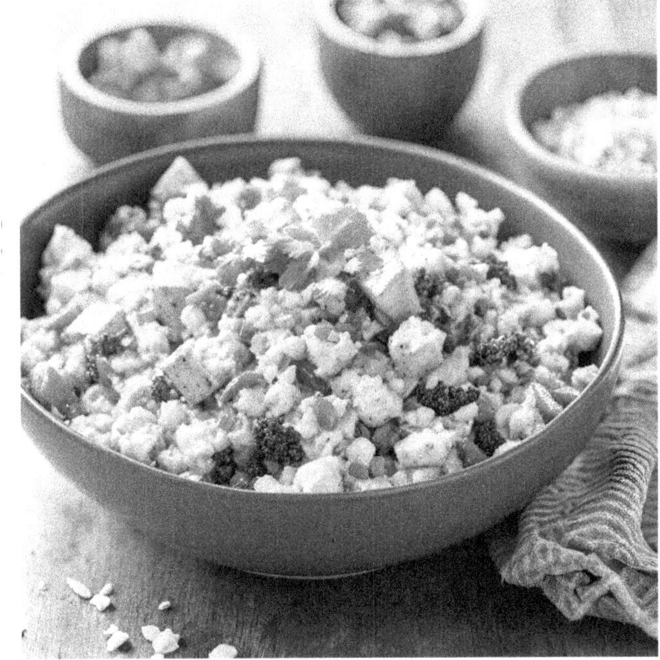

18. Peanut Butter and Jelly Oatmeal

Ingredients:

- 1 cup rolled oats
- 2 cups water
- 1/2 cup low-fat milk
- 2 tablespoons natural peanut butter
- 2 tablespoons fruit preserves or jam (no added sugar)
- 1/2 teaspoon cinnamon
- 1 tablespoon chia seeds

Instructions:

1. In a medium saucepan, bring water to a boil. Add the rolled oats and reduce heat to a simmer.
2. Cook the oats, stirring occasionally, until the water is absorbed, about 5-7 minutes.
3. Stir in the milk, peanut butter, cinnamon, and chia seeds. Continue to cook until the oats are creamy, about 2-3 more minutes.
4. Divide the oatmeal into bowls and swirl in the fruit preserves or jam.
5. Serve immediately.

Nutrition Info per Serving:

- Calories: 350
- Protein: 10g
- Carbohydrates: 50g
- Fat: 15g
- Fiber: 8g
- Sugar: 12g

Number of Servings:

- **2 servings**

Cooking Time:

- **15 minutes**

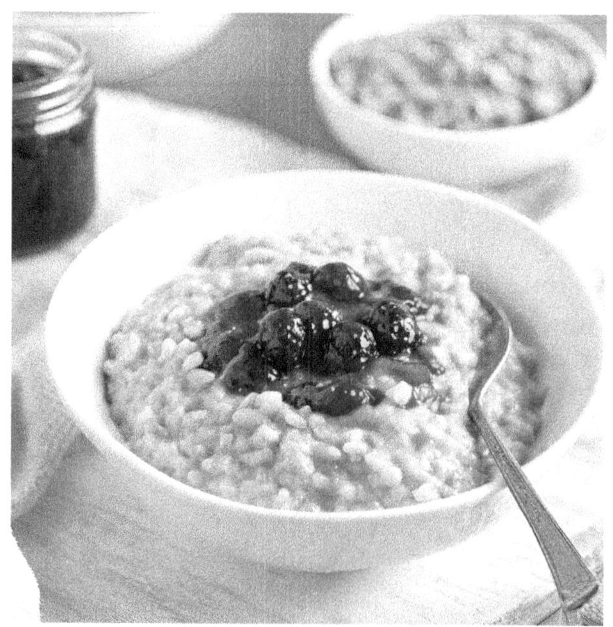

19. Broccoli and Cheese Frittata

Ingredients:

- 6 large eggs
- 1/4 cup low-fat milk
- 1 cup steamed broccoli florets
- 1/2 cup shredded low-fat cheddar cheese
- 1/4 cup diced onion
- 1 tablespoon olive oil
- 1/4 teaspoon garlic powder
- 1/4 teaspoon black pepper

Instructions:

1. Preheat the oven to 350°F (175°C).
2. In a medium bowl, whisk together the eggs and milk until well combined.
3. Heat olive oil in an oven-safe skillet over medium heat.
4. Add the onion and cook until softened, about 3 minutes.
5. Add the steamed broccoli and cook for another 2 minutes.
6. Pour the egg mixture over the vegetables in the skillet. Sprinkle with garlic powder and black pepper.
7. Cook on the stovetop for 2-3 minutes, until the edges start to set.
8. Sprinkle the shredded cheese over the top.
9. Transfer the skillet to the oven and bake for 15-20 minutes, or until the frittata is fully set and golden.
10. Let cool slightly before slicing and serving.

Nutrition Info per Serving:

- Calories: 200
- Protein: 15g
- Carbohydrates: 5g
- Fat: 13g
- Fiber: 1g
- Sugar: 2g

Number of Servings:

- **4 servings**

Cooking Time:

- **25 minutes**

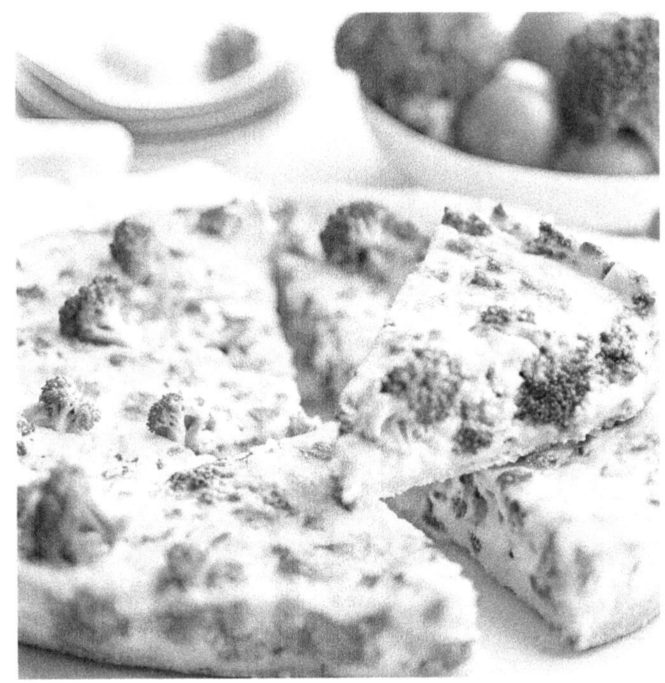

20. Pear and Walnut Oatmeal

Ingredients:

- 1 cup rolled oats
- 2 cups water
- 1/2 cup low-fat milk
- 1 ripe pear, diced
- 1/4 cup chopped walnuts
- 1 tablespoon honey or maple syrup
- 1/2 teaspoon ground cinnamon

Instructions:

1. In a medium saucepan, bring water to a boil. Add the rolled oats and reduce heat to a simmer.
2. Cook the oats, stirring occasionally, until the water is absorbed, about 5-7 minutes.
3. Stir in the milk, diced pear, honey or maple syrup, and cinnamon. Continue to cook until the oats are creamy and the pear is tender, about 2-3 more minutes.
4. Divide the oatmeal into bowls and top with chopped walnuts.
5. Serve immediately.

Nutrition Info per Serving:

- Calories: 300
- Protein: 8g
- Carbohydrates: 50g
- Fat: 10g
- Fiber: 7g
- Sugar: 15g

Number of Servings:

- **2 servings**

Cooking Time:

- **15 minutes**

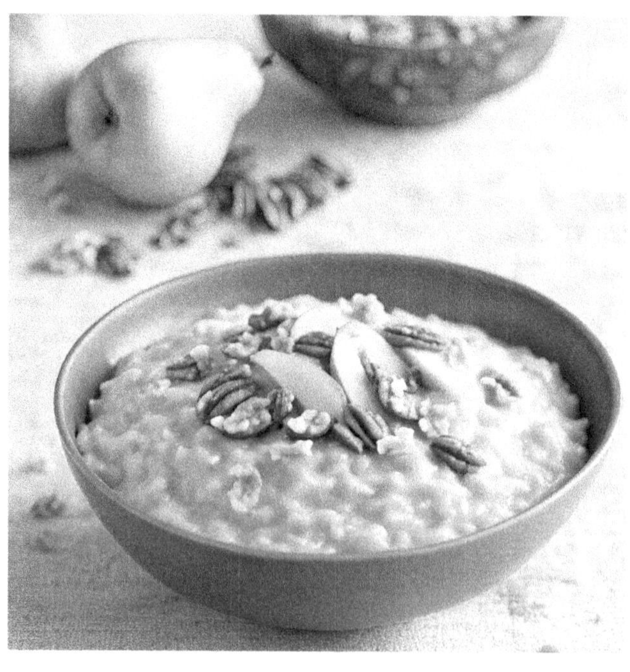

21. Vegetable and Quinoa Breakfast Bowl

Ingredients:

- 1 cup quinoa
- 2 cups water
- 1 tablespoon olive oil
- 1 cup diced bell pepper
- 1 cup chopped spinach
- 1/2 cup diced zucchini
- 1/4 cup diced onion
- 1/4 teaspoon garlic powder
- 1/4 teaspoon cumin
- 1/4 teaspoon black pepper
- 2 tablespoons chopped fresh parsley (optional, for garnish)

Instructions:

1. Rinse the quinoa under cold water.
2. In a medium saucepan, bring water to a boil. Add the quinoa, reduce heat to low, and cover. Simmer for 15 minutes, or until the water is absorbed and the quinoa is tender.
3. Meanwhile, heat olive oil in a large skillet over medium heat.
4. Add the onion and cook until translucent, about 3 minutes.
5. Add the bell pepper and zucchini, and cook until tender, about 5 minutes.
6. Add the spinach, garlic powder, cumin, and black pepper. Cook until the spinach is wilted, about 2-3 minutes.
7. Divide the cooked quinoa into bowls and top with the vegetable mixture.
8. Garnish with fresh parsley if desired.
9. Serve immediately.

Nutrition Info per Serving:

- Calories: 250
- Protein: 8g
- Carbohydrates: 40g
- Fat: 8g
- Fiber: 5g
- Sugar: 5g

Number of Servings:

- **4 servings**

Cooking Time:

- **25 minutes**

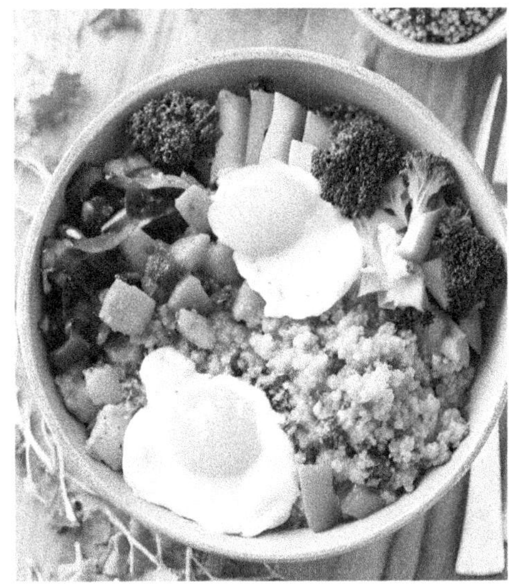

22. Almond Flour Blueberry Muffins

Ingredients:

- 2 cups almond flour
- 1/2 teaspoon baking soda
- 1/2 teaspoon ground cinnamon
- 3 large eggs
- 1/4 cup honey or maple syrup
- 1/4 cup unsweetened almond milk
- 1 teaspoon vanilla extract
- 1 cup fresh or frozen blueberries

Instructions:

1. Preheat the oven to 350°F (175°C) and line a muffin tin with paper liners.
2. In a large bowl, mix together the almond flour, baking soda, and cinnamon.
3. In another bowl, whisk together the eggs, honey or maple syrup, almond milk, and vanilla extract.
4. Pour the wet ingredients into the dry ingredients and mix until well combined.
5. Gently fold in the blueberries.
6. Divide the batter evenly among the muffin cups.
7. Bake for 20-25 minutes, or until a toothpick inserted into the center comes out clean.
8. Allow the muffins to cool in the pan for 10 minutes, then transfer to a wire rack to cool completely.

Nutrition Info per Serving:

- Calories: 180
- Protein: 6g
- Carbohydrates: 12g
- Fat: 12g
- Fiber: 3g
- Sugar: 8g

Number of Servings:

- **12 muffins**

Cooking Time:

- **25 minutes**

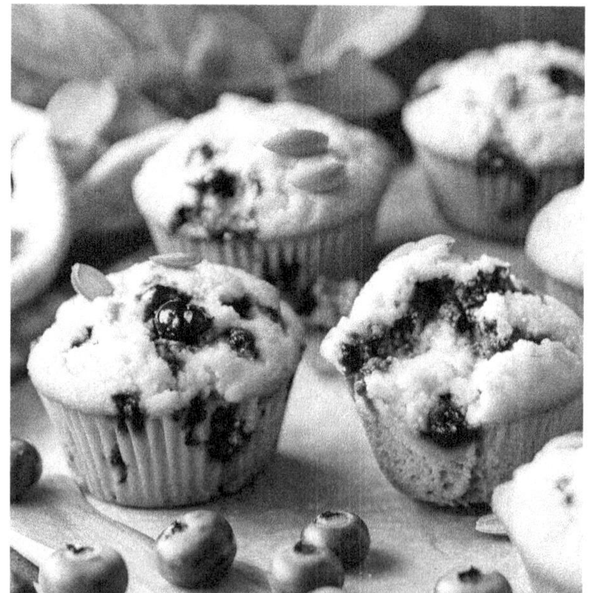

23. Egg White and Avocado Wrap

Ingredients:

- 4 large egg whites
- 1 ripe avocado, sliced
- 1/4 cup diced tomatoes
- 1/4 cup diced onion
- 1/4 cup chopped spinach
- 1 teaspoon olive oil
- 1/4 teaspoon garlic powder
- 4 whole wheat tortillas

Instructions:

1. Heat the olive oil in a non-stick skillet over medium heat.
2. Add the onions and cook until translucent, about 3 minutes.
3. Add the tomatoes and spinach, and cook for another 2 minutes.
4. Pour the egg whites into the skillet and sprinkle with garlic powder. Cook, stirring gently, until the egg whites are set, about 3-4 minutes.
5. Warm the tortillas in a separate skillet or microwave.
6. Divide the egg white mixture among the tortillas, top with avocado slices, and wrap tightly.
7. Serve immediately.

Nutrition Info per Serving:

- Calories: 250
- Protein: 10g
- Carbohydrates: 30g
- Fat: 10g
- Fiber: 6g
- Sugar: 3g

Number of Servings:

- **4 wraps**

Cooking Time:

- **15 minutes**

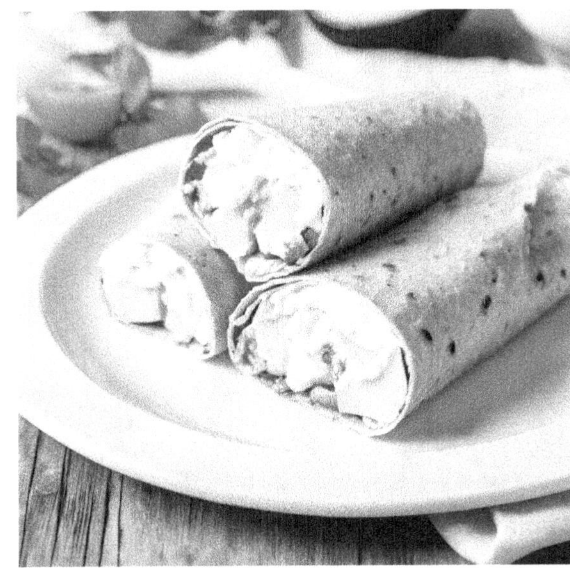

24. Sweet Corn and Zucchini Pancakes
Ingredients:
- 1 cup grated zucchini
- 1 cup corn kernels (fresh or frozen)
- 1/2 cup whole wheat flour
- 1/4 cup cornmeal
- 1/2 teaspoon baking powder
- 1/4 teaspoon paprika
- 1/4 teaspoon cumin
- 1/4 cup unsweetened almond milk
- 1 large egg
- 1 tablespoon olive oil (for cooking)

Instructions:
1. In a large bowl, combine the grated zucchini, corn kernels, whole wheat flour, cornmeal, baking powder, paprika, and cumin.
2. In a separate bowl, whisk together the almond milk and egg.
3. Pour the wet ingredients into the dry ingredients and mix until well combined.
4. Heat the olive oil in a non-stick skillet over medium heat.
5. Drop 1/4 cup of batter into the skillet for each pancake. Cook until bubbles form on the surface and the edges look set, about 2-3 minutes.
6. Flip the pancakes and cook for an additional 2-3 minutes, until golden brown.
7. Serve immediately.

Nutrition Info per Serving:
- Calories: 150
- Protein: 5g
- Carbohydrates: 20g
- Fat: 5g
- Fiber: 3g
- Sugar: 3g

Number of Servings:
- **4 servings (8 pancakes)**

Cooking Time:
- **20 minutes**

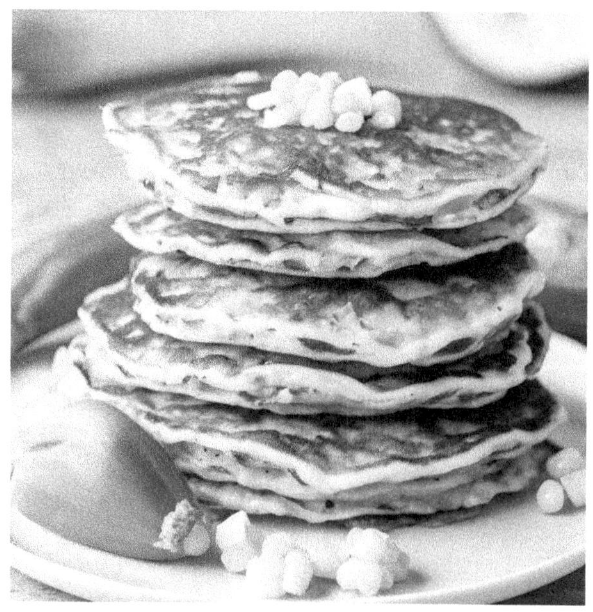

25. Raspberry Chia Jam on Toast

Ingredients:

- 2 cups fresh or frozen raspberries
- 2 tablespoons chia seeds
- 1 tablespoon honey or maple syrup
- 8 slices whole grain bread

Instructions:

1. In a medium saucepan, heat the raspberries over medium heat until they break down, about 5 minutes.
2. Stir in the chia seeds and honey or maple syrup. Cook for an additional 5 minutes, until the mixture thickens.
3. Remove from heat and let the jam cool to room temperature.
4. Toast the whole grain bread slices.
5. Spread the raspberry chia jam over the toast.
6. Serve immediately.

Nutrition Info per Serving:

- Calories: 180
- Protein: 5g
- Carbohydrates: 30g
- Fat: 4g
- Fiber: 7g
- Sugar: 8g

Number of Servings:

- **4 servings (2 slices of toast each)**

Cooking Time:

- **10 minutes**

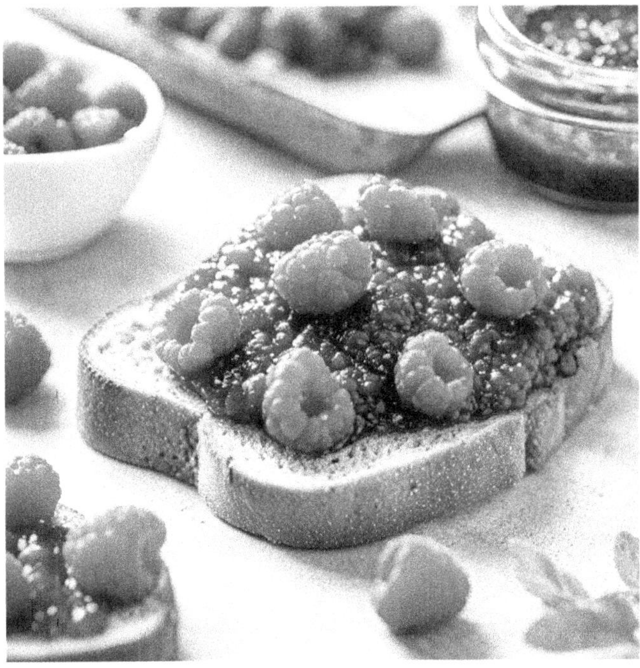

26. Soy Yogurt with Compote

Ingredients:

- 2 cups plain soy yogurt
- 1 cup mixed berries (blueberries, strawberries, raspberries)
- 1 tablespoon honey or maple syrup
- 1/2 teaspoon vanilla extract
- 1 tablespoon chia seeds

Instructions:

1. In a small saucepan, combine the mixed berries and honey or maple syrup. Cook over medium heat until the berries break down and the mixture thickens, about 5-7 minutes.
2. Stir in the vanilla extract and chia seeds. Remove from heat and let cool slightly.
3. Divide the soy yogurt into bowls.
4. Top each bowl with the berry compote.
5. Serve immediately.

Nutrition Info per Serving:

- Calories: 180
- Protein: 6g
- Carbohydrates: 25g
- Fat: 6g
- Fiber: 5g
- Sugar: 15g

Number of Servings:

- **2 servings**

Cooking Time:

- **10 minutes**

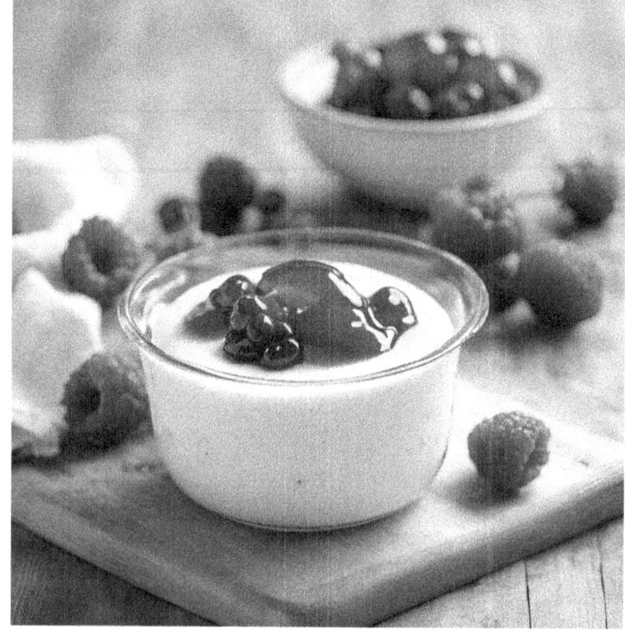

Vegetables

1. Roasted Cauliflower Steaks

Ingredients:

- 1 large cauliflower head, sliced into 1-inch thick steaks
- 2 tablespoons olive oil
- 1 teaspoon garlic powder
- 1 teaspoon paprika
- 1/2 teaspoon turmeric
- 1/4 teaspoon black pepper
- 1 tablespoon chopped fresh parsley (optional, for garnish)

Instructions:

1. Preheat the oven to 425°F (220°C) and line a baking sheet with parchment paper.
2. Place the cauliflower steaks on the prepared baking sheet.
3. In a small bowl, mix together the olive oil, garlic powder, paprika, turmeric, and black pepper.
4. Brush the mixture over both sides of the cauliflower steaks.
5. Roast in the preheated oven for 25-30 minutes, flipping halfway through, until the cauliflower is tender and golden brown.
6. Garnish with fresh parsley, if desired, and serve immediately.

Nutrition Info per Serving:

- Calories: 120
- Protein: 3g
- Carbohydrates: 8g
- Fat: 9g
- Fiber: 4g
- Sugar: 2g

Number of Servings:

- **4 servings**

Cooking Time:

- **30 minutes**

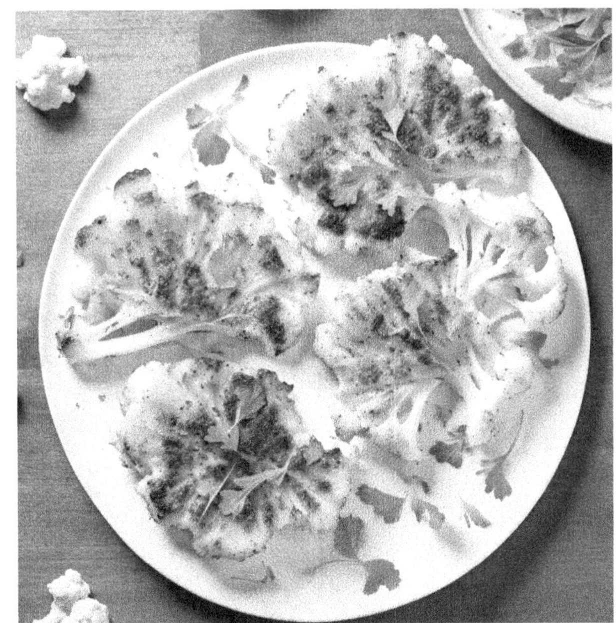

2. Stuffed Bell Peppers

Ingredients:

- 4 large bell peppers, tops cut off and seeds removed
- 1 cup cooked quinoa
- 1 cup black beans, rinsed and drained
- 1 cup corn kernels (fresh or frozen)
- 1/2 cup diced tomatoes
- 1/2 cup diced onion
- 1 tablespoon olive oil
- 1 teaspoon cumin
- 1 teaspoon chili powder
- 1/4 teaspoon black pepper
- 1/4 cup shredded low-fat cheese (optional)
- Fresh cilantro for garnish (optional)

Instructions:

1. Preheat the oven to 375°F (190°C).
2. In a large skillet, heat the olive oil over medium heat. Add the onion and cook until softened, about 5 minutes.
3. Add the diced tomatoes, black beans, corn, cooked quinoa, cumin, chili powder, and black pepper. Cook for another 5 minutes, stirring occasionally.
4. Stuff the bell peppers with the quinoa mixture and place them in a baking dish.
5. Cover with aluminum foil and bake for 30 minutes.
6. Remove the foil, sprinkle with cheese (if using), and bake for an additional 10 minutes, until the peppers are tender and the cheese is melted.
7. Garnish with fresh cilantro, if desired, and serve immediately.

Nutrition Info per Serving:

- Calories: 220
- Protein: 8g
- Carbohydrates: 35g
- Fat: 7g
- Fiber: 8g
- Sugar: 7g

Number of Servings:

- 4 servings

Cooking Time:

- 40 minutes

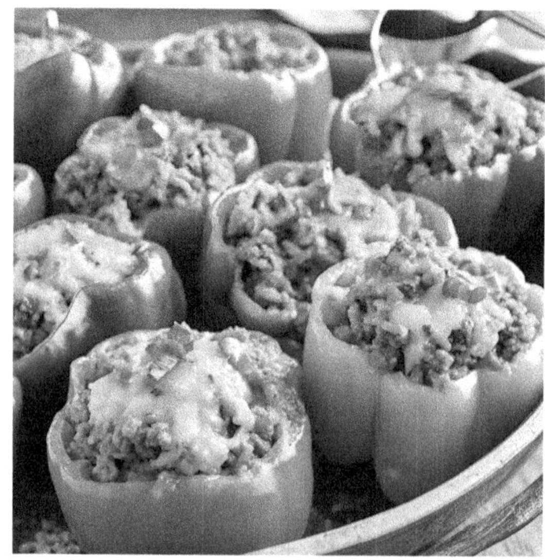

3. Grilled Zucchini Rolls

Ingredients:

- 2 large zucchinis, sliced lengthwise into thin strips
- 1 tablespoon olive oil
- 1/2 cup low-fat ricotta cheese
- 1/4 cup chopped fresh basil
- 1/4 teaspoon garlic powder
- 1/4 teaspoon black pepper
- 1/2 cup marinara sauce (for serving)

Instructions:

1. Preheat a grill or grill pan over medium heat.
2. Brush the zucchini slices with olive oil on both sides.
3. Grill the zucchini slices for 2-3 minutes per side, until tender and grill marks appear.
4. In a small bowl, mix the ricotta cheese, fresh basil, garlic powder, and black pepper.
5. Place a spoonful of the ricotta mixture at one end of each zucchini slice and roll up.
6. Serve the zucchini rolls with warmed marinara sauce.

Nutrition Info per Serving:

- Calories: 130
- Protein: 6g
- Carbohydrates: 7g
- Fat: 9g
- Fiber: 2g
- Sugar: 3g

Number of Servings:

- **4 servings**

Cooking Time:

- **15 minutes**

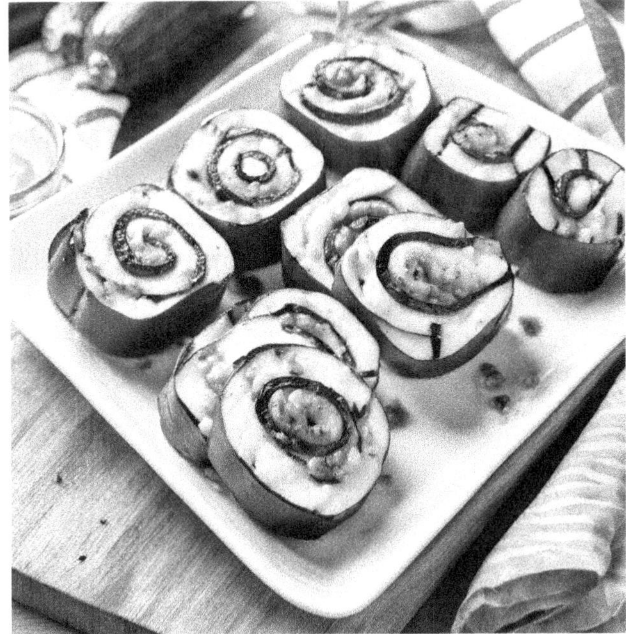

4. Spaghetti Squash Primavera

Ingredients:

- 1 large spaghetti squash
- 2 tablespoons olive oil
- 1 cup cherry tomatoes, halved
- 1 cup broccoli florets
- 1 cup diced bell pepper
- 1/2 cup sliced mushrooms
- 1/2 cup diced onion
- 2 cloves garlic, minced
- 1 teaspoon dried oregano
- 1/4 teaspoon black pepper
- 1/4 cup grated Parmesan cheese (optional)
- Fresh basil for garnish (optional)

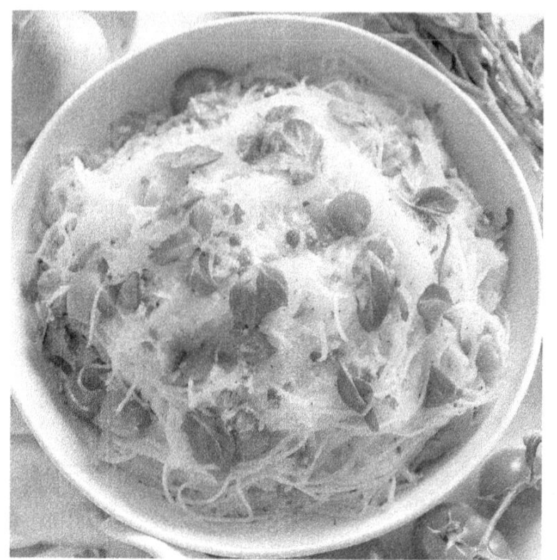

Instructions:

1. Preheat the oven to 400°F (200°C) and line a baking sheet with parchment paper.
2. Cut the spaghetti squash in half lengthwise and remove the seeds. Drizzle with 1 tablespoon of olive oil and place cut side down on the baking sheet.
3. Roast in the preheated oven for 40 minutes, or until the squash is tender.
4. While the squash is roasting, heat the remaining 1 tablespoon of olive oil in a large skillet over medium heat. Add the onion and garlic, and cook until fragrant, about 3 minutes.
5. Add the cherry tomatoes, broccoli, bell pepper, and mushrooms. Cook for 5-7 minutes, until the vegetables are tender.
6. Stir in the dried oregano and black pepper.
7. Once the squash is cooked, use a fork to scrape out the flesh into spaghetti-like strands and add it to the skillet with the vegetables. Toss to combine.
8. Sprinkle with Parmesan cheese if desired and garnish with fresh basil.
9. Serve immediately.

Nutrition Info per Serving:

- Calories: 180
- Protein: 5g
- Carbohydrates: 25g
- Fat: 8g
- Fiber: 6g
- Sugar: 8g

Number of Servings:

- **4 servings**

Cooking Time:

- **45 minutes**

5. Eggplant Parmesan

Ingredients:

- 2 large eggplants, sliced into 1/4-inch rounds
- 2 tablespoons olive oil
- 1 cup whole wheat breadcrumbs
- 1/2 cup grated Parmesan cheese
- 1 teaspoon dried oregano
- 1 teaspoon garlic powder
- 1/4 teaspoon black pepper
- 1 1/2 cups marinara sauce
- 1 cup shredded low-fat mozzarella cheese
- Fresh basil for garnish (optional)

Instructions:

1. Preheat the oven to 375°F (190°C). Line a baking sheet with parchment paper.
2. Brush both sides of the eggplant slices with olive oil and place on the prepared baking sheet.
3. In a shallow bowl, combine the breadcrumbs, Parmesan cheese, oregano, garlic powder, and black pepper.
4. Press each eggplant slice into the breadcrumb mixture, coating both sides.
5. Bake the eggplant slices for 20 minutes, flipping halfway through, until golden and tender.
6. In a baking dish, spread 1/2 cup of marinara sauce. Layer half of the eggplant slices over the sauce.
7. Top with another 1/2 cup of marinara sauce and half of the mozzarella cheese.
8. Repeat with the remaining eggplant slices, marinara sauce, and mozzarella cheese.
9. Bake for 20-25 minutes, until the cheese is melted and bubbly.
10. Garnish with fresh basil if desired and serve immediately.

Nutrition Info per Serving:

- Calories: 250
- Protein: 12g
- Carbohydrates: 30g
- Fat: 12g
- Fiber: 8g
- Sugar: 10g

Number of Servings:

- 4 servings

Cooking Time:

- 45 minutes

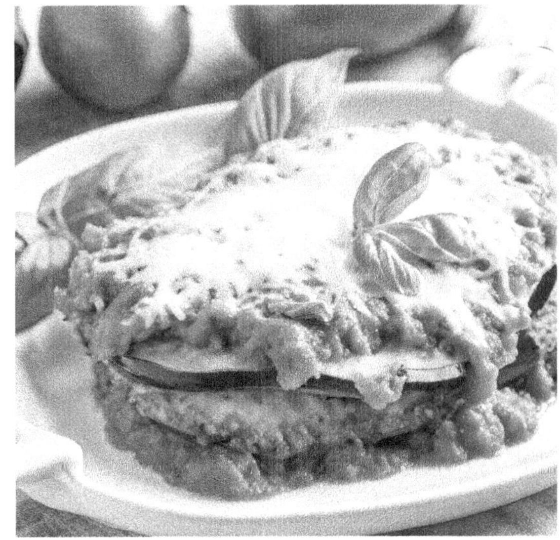

6. Kale Salad with Avocado and Nuts

Ingredients:

- 4 cups chopped kale
- 1 ripe avocado, diced
- 1/4 cup chopped walnuts
- 1/4 cup dried cranberries
- 1 tablespoon olive oil
- 1 tablespoon lemon juice
- 1/4 teaspoon garlic powder
- 1/4 teaspoon black pepper

Instructions:

1. In a large bowl, massage the chopped kale with the olive oil, lemon juice, garlic powder, and black pepper until the kale is tender, about 2-3 minutes.
2. Add the diced avocado, chopped walnuts, and dried cranberries to the bowl.
3. Toss to combine.
4. Serve immediately.

Nutrition Info per Serving:

- Calories: 220
- Protein: 5g
- Carbohydrates: 18g
- Fat: 16g
- Fiber: 7g
- Sugar: 7g

Number of Servings:

- **4 servings**

Cooking Time:

- **10 minutes**

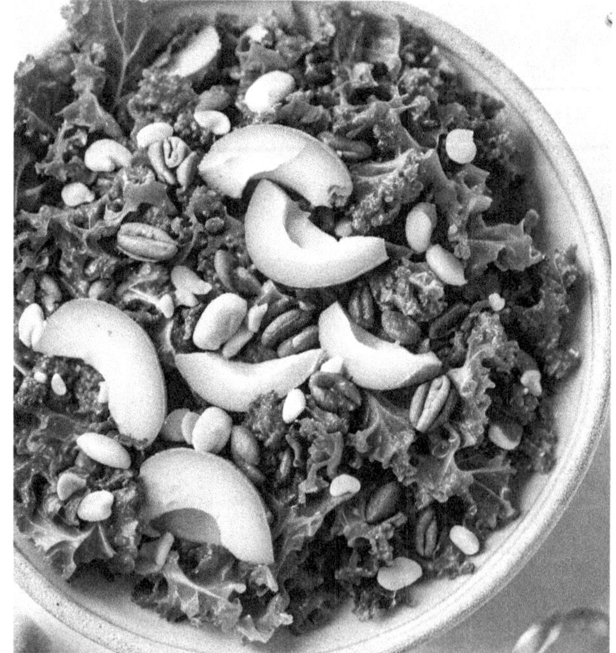

7. Vegetable Stir-Fry

Ingredients:

- 1 tablespoon olive oil
- 1 cup broccoli florets
- 1 cup sliced bell peppers (red, yellow, green)
- 1 cup sliced carrots
- 1/2 cup snow peas
- 1/2 cup sliced mushrooms
- 1/4 cup diced onion
- 2 cloves garlic, minced
- 1 tablespoon low-sodium soy sauce
- 1 teaspoon grated fresh ginger
- 1/4 teaspoon black pepper

Instructions:

1. Heat the olive oil in a large skillet or wok over medium-high heat.
2. Add the onion and garlic, and sauté for 2 minutes until fragrant.
3. Add the broccoli, bell peppers, carrots, snow peas, and mushrooms. Stir-fry for 5-7 minutes, until the vegetables are tender-crisp.
4. Stir in the soy sauce, ginger, and black pepper. Cook for an additional 2 minutes.
5. Serve immediately.

Nutrition Info per Serving:

- Calories: 120
- Protein: 4g
- Carbohydrates: 18g
- Fat: 5g
- Fiber: 5g
- Sugar: 7g

Number of Servings:

- **4 servings**

Cooking Time:

- **15 minutes**

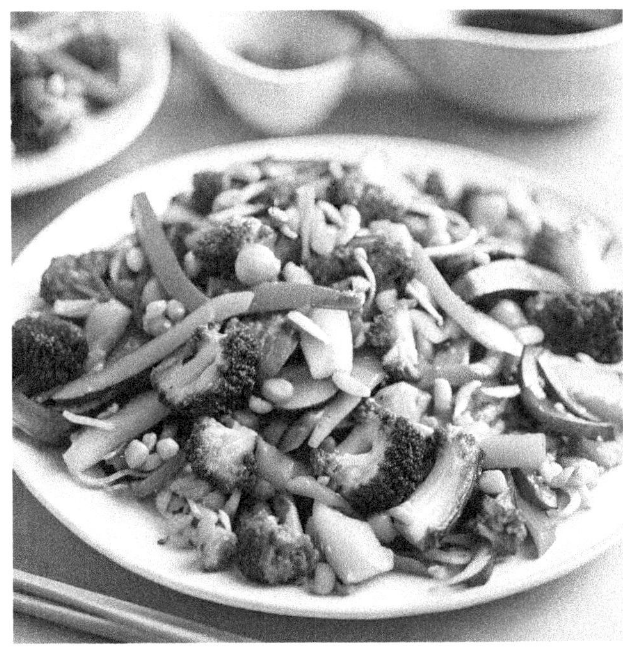

8. Roasted Brussels Sprouts with Garlic

Ingredients:

- 1 pound Brussels sprouts, trimmed and halved
- 2 tablespoons olive oil
- 3 cloves garlic, minced
- 1/4 teaspoon black pepper
- 1 tablespoon balsamic vinegar (optional)

Instructions:

1. Preheat the oven to 400°F (200°C) and line a baking sheet with parchment paper.
2. In a large bowl, toss the Brussels sprouts with olive oil, garlic, and black pepper.
3. Spread the Brussels sprouts in a single layer on the prepared baking sheet.
4. Roast for 20-25 minutes, stirring halfway through, until the Brussels sprouts are tender and golden brown.
5. Drizzle with balsamic vinegar if desired.
6. Serve immediately.

Nutrition Info per Serving:

- Calories: 150
- Protein: 4g
- Carbohydrates: 14g
- Fat: 10g
- Fiber: 5g
- Sugar: 3g

Number of Servings:

- **4 servings**

Cooking Time:

- **25 minutes**

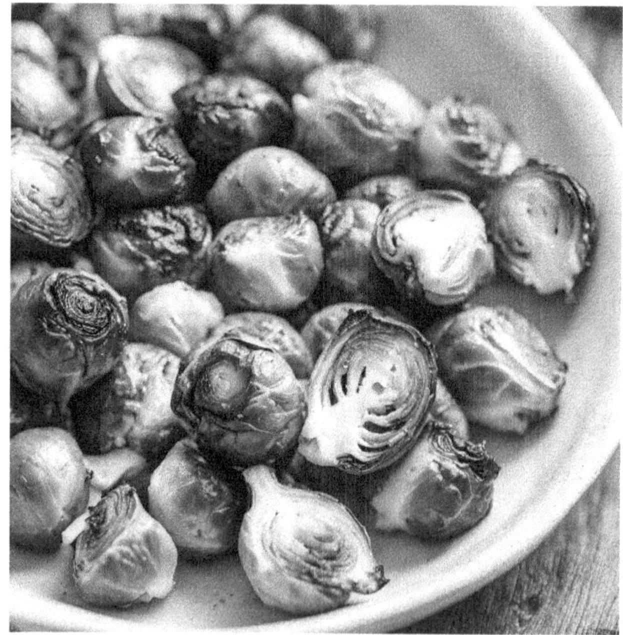

9. Butternut Squash Risotto

Ingredients:

- 1 cup Arborio rice
- 4 cups low-sodium vegetable broth
- 1 tablespoon olive oil
- 1 cup diced onion
- 2 cloves garlic, minced
- 2 cups diced butternut squash
- 1/4 cup grated Parmesan cheese (optional)
- 1/4 teaspoon black pepper
- Fresh thyme for garnish (optional)

Instructions:

1. In a medium saucepan, heat the vegetable broth over low heat.
2. In a large skillet, heat the olive oil over medium heat. Add the onion and garlic, and cook until softened, about 3-4 minutes.
3. Add the diced butternut squash and cook for another 5 minutes, stirring occasionally.
4. Add the Arborio rice to the skillet and cook, stirring frequently, for 2 minutes until the rice is lightly toasted.
5. Begin adding the warm broth to the rice mixture, one ladle at a time, stirring constantly. Wait until the broth is mostly absorbed before adding more. Continue this process until the rice is creamy and cooked through, about 20 minutes.
6. Stir in the Parmesan cheese (if using) and black pepper.
7. Garnish with fresh thyme if desired.
8. Serve immediately.

Nutrition Info per Serving:

- Calories: 250
- Protein: 5g
- Carbohydrates: 50g
- Fat: 5g
- Fiber: 4g
- Sugar: 3g

Number of Servings:

- **4 servings**

Cooking Time:

- **30 minutes**

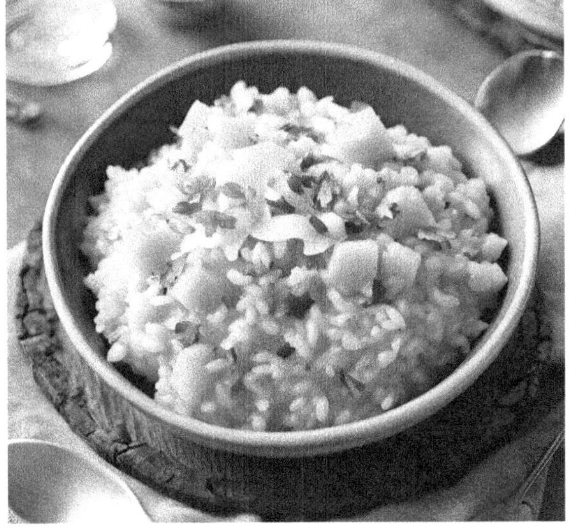

10. Mushroom Stroganoff

Ingredients:

- 2 tablespoons olive oil
- 1 large onion, diced
- 3 cloves garlic, minced
- 1 pound mushrooms, sliced
- 1 teaspoon paprika
- 1/2 teaspoon dried thyme
- 1/4 teaspoon black pepper
- 1 tablespoon all-purpose flour
- 1 cup low-sodium vegetable broth
- 1/2 cup unsweetened almond milk
- 1 tablespoon Dijon mustard
- 1 tablespoon soy sauce
- 1/4 cup chopped fresh parsley (optional, for garnish)
- Cooked whole wheat pasta or brown rice (for serving)

Instructions:

1. Heat olive oil in a large skillet over medium heat. Add the onion and cook until softened, about 5 minutes.
2. Add the garlic and cook for another minute until fragrant.
3. Add the mushrooms, paprika, thyme, and black pepper. Cook until the mushrooms release their juices and are tender, about 10 minutes.
4. Sprinkle the flour over the mushroom mixture and stir well to combine. Cook for 1-2 minutes.
5. Gradually add the vegetable broth, stirring constantly to prevent lumps. Bring to a simmer.
6. Stir in the almond milk, Dijon mustard, and soy sauce. Cook for another 5 minutes until the sauce thickens.
7. Serve over cooked whole wheat pasta or brown rice. Garnish with chopped parsley if desired.

Nutrition Info per Serving:

- Calories: 200
- Protein: 5g
- Carbohydrates: 15g
- Fat: 12g
- Fiber: 3g
- Sugar: 5g

Number of Servings:

- **4 servings**

Cooking Time:

- **25 minutes**

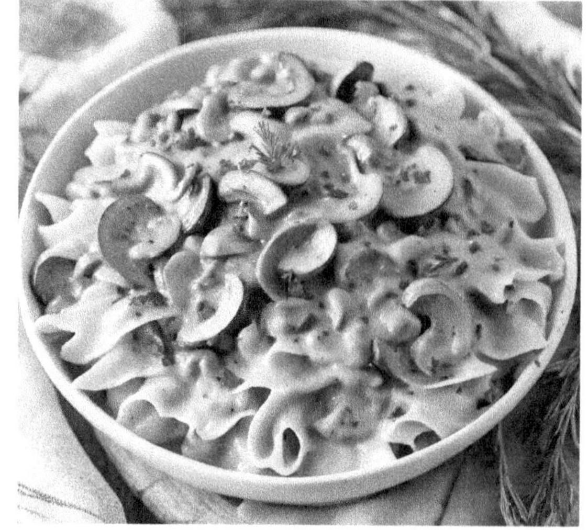

11. Green Beans Almondine

Ingredients:

- 1 pound fresh green beans, trimmed
- 2 tablespoons olive oil
- 1/4 cup sliced almonds
- 2 cloves garlic, minced
- 1 tablespoon lemon juice
- 1/4 teaspoon black pepper

Instructions:

1. Bring a large pot of water to a boil. Add the green beans and cook for 3-4 minutes until tender-crisp. Drain and rinse under cold water to stop the cooking process.
2. Heat olive oil in a large skillet over medium heat. Add the sliced almonds and cook until golden brown, about 3 minutes.
3. Add the garlic and cook for another minute until fragrant.
4. Add the green beans to the skillet and toss to coat in the almond mixture. Cook for another 2-3 minutes until heated through.
5. Stir in the lemon juice and black pepper.
6. Serve immediately.

Nutrition Info per Serving:

- Calories: 120
- Protein: 3g
- Carbohydrates: 10g
- Fat: 9g
- Fiber: 4g
- Sugar: 3g

Number of Servings:

- **4 servings**

Cooking Time:

- **10 minutes**

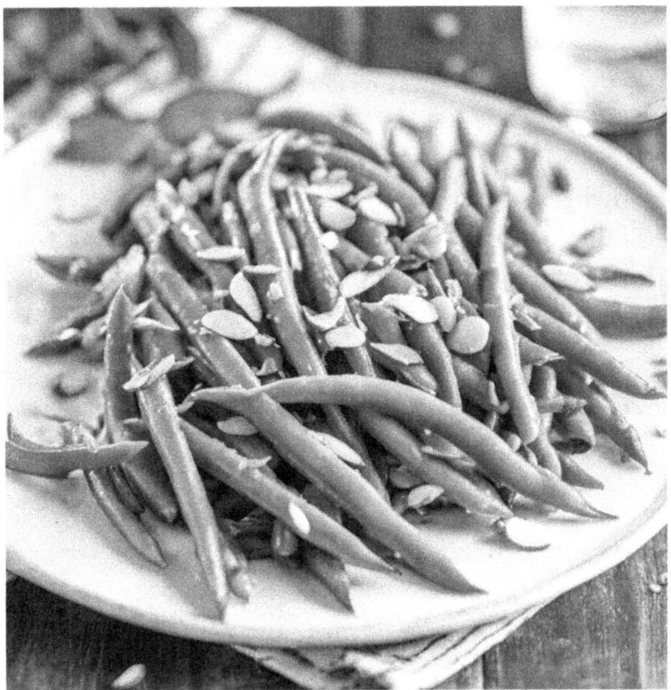

12. Cucumber Gazpacho

Ingredients:

- 2 large cucumbers, peeled and chopped
- 1 green bell pepper, chopped
- 2 cloves garlic, minced
- 1/4 cup chopped fresh parsley
- 1/4 cup chopped fresh dill
- 2 tablespoons olive oil
- 2 tablespoons white wine vinegar
- 1/4 teaspoon black pepper
- 1 cup cold water
- 1 cup plain Greek yogurt (optional, for garnish)

Instructions:

1. In a blender, combine the cucumbers, green bell pepper, garlic, parsley, dill, olive oil, white wine vinegar, and black pepper. Blend until smooth.
2. Add cold water to achieve the desired consistency and blend again.
3. Chill in the refrigerator for at least 1 hour before serving.
4. Serve cold, garnished with a dollop of Greek yogurt if desired.

Nutrition Info per Serving:

- Calories: 100
- Protein: 2g
- Carbohydrates: 7g
- Fat: 7g
- Fiber: 2g
- Sugar: 4g

Number of Servings:

- 4 servings

Cooking Time:

- 10 minutes (plus 1 hour chilling)

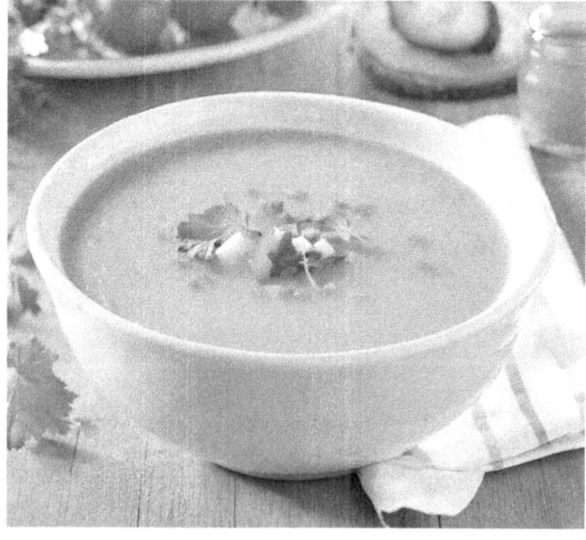

13. Lentil and Vegetable Stew

Ingredients:

- 2 tablespoons olive oil
- 1 large onion, diced
- 3 cloves garlic, minced
- 2 carrots, chopped
- 2 celery stalks, chopped
- 1 zucchini, chopped
- 1 cup dried green or brown lentils, rinsed
- 4 cups low-sodium vegetable broth
- 1 can (14.5 ounces) diced tomatoes
- 1 teaspoon dried thyme
- 1 teaspoon ground cumin
- 1/4 teaspoon black pepper
- 2 cups chopped kale or spinach

Instructions:

1. Heat olive oil in a large pot over medium heat. Add the onion and cook until softened, about 5 minutes.
2. Add the garlic, carrots, celery, and zucchini. Cook for another 5 minutes until the vegetables begin to soften.
3. Stir in the lentils, vegetable broth, diced tomatoes, thyme, cumin, and black pepper. Bring to a boil.
4. Reduce heat to low and simmer for 30-35 minutes, until the lentils are tender.
5. Stir in the kale or spinach and cook for an additional 5 minutes until wilted.
6. Serve immediately.

Nutrition Info per Serving:

- Calories: 250
- Protein: 10g
- Carbohydrates: 35g
- Fat: 8g
- Fiber: 12g
- Sugar: 8g

Number of Servings:

- **4 servings**

Cooking Time:

- **45 minutes**

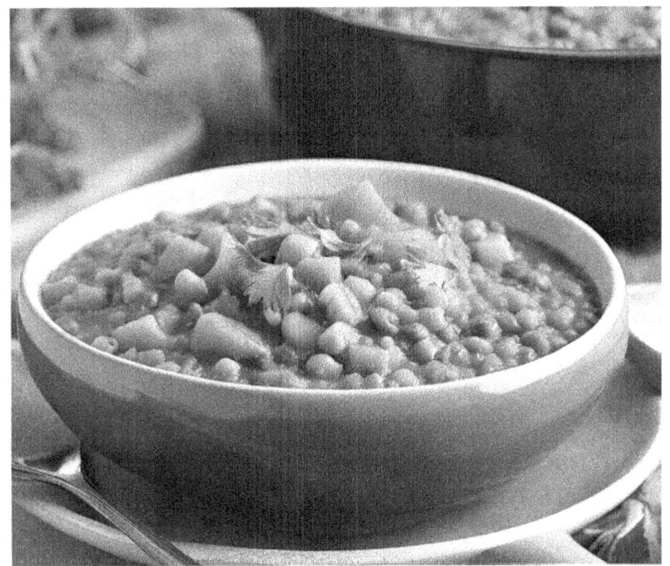

14. Vegan Cabbage Rolls

Ingredients:

- 1 large head of cabbage
- 1 cup cooked quinoa
- 1 can (15 ounces) black beans, rinsed and drained
- 1 cup diced tomatoes
- 1/2 cup diced onion
- 2 cloves garlic, minced
- 1 teaspoon ground cumin
- 1 teaspoon smoked paprika
- 1/4 teaspoon black pepper
- 1 tablespoon olive oil
- 2 cups tomato sauce

Instructions:

1. Preheat the oven to 350°F (175°C).
2. Bring a large pot of water to a boil. Carefully remove 12 large leaves from the cabbage head and blanch in the boiling water for 2-3 minutes until pliable. Remove and drain.
3. In a large skillet, heat the olive oil over medium heat. Add the onion and garlic, and cook until softened, about 5 minutes.
4. Add the diced tomatoes, black beans, quinoa, cumin, smoked paprika, and black pepper. Cook for another 5 minutes until well combined and heated through.
5. Lay a cabbage leaf flat and place about 1/4 cup of the filling mixture in the center. Roll up, tucking in the sides to form a neat roll. Repeat with remaining cabbage leaves and filling.
6. Spread 1 cup of tomato sauce in the bottom of a baking dish. Place the cabbage rolls seam side down in the dish. Pour the remaining tomato sauce over the top.
7. Cover with aluminum foil and bake for 30 minutes.
8. Remove the foil and bake for an additional 10 minutes.
9. Serve immediately.

Nutrition Info per Serving:

- Calories: 200
- Protein: 7g
- Carbohydrates: 35g
- Fat: 5g
- Fiber: 10g
- Sugar: 10g

Number of Servings:

- **4 servings (3 rolls each)**

Cooking Time:

- **50 minutes**

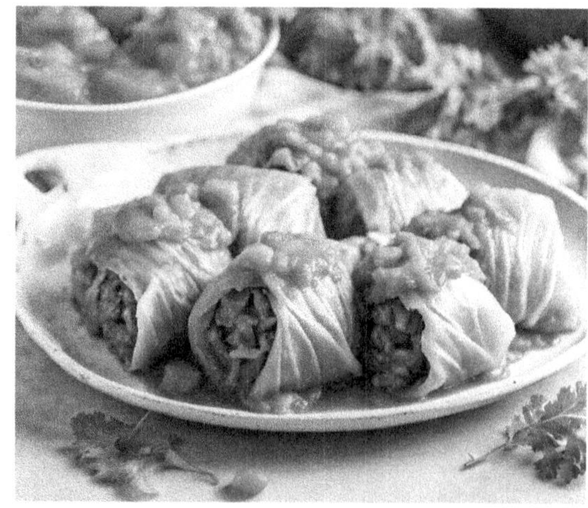

15. Curried Cauliflower Soup

Ingredients:

- 1 large cauliflower head, chopped into florets
- 1 large onion, diced
- 3 cloves garlic, minced
- 1 tablespoon olive oil
- 1 tablespoon curry powder
- 1 teaspoon ground turmeric
- 1/4 teaspoon black pepper
- 4 cups low-sodium vegetable broth
- 1 cup unsweetened coconut milk
- Fresh cilantro for garnish (optional)

Instructions:

1. Heat olive oil in a large pot over medium heat. Add the onion and garlic, and cook until softened, about 5 minutes.
2. Add the curry powder, turmeric, and black pepper, and cook for another minute until fragrant.
3. Add the cauliflower florets and vegetable broth. Bring to a boil, then reduce heat and simmer for 20 minutes, until the cauliflower is tender.
4. Using an immersion blender, blend the soup until smooth. Alternatively, transfer the soup to a blender and blend in batches.
5. Stir in the coconut milk and heat through.
6. Serve garnished with fresh cilantro if desired.

Nutrition Info per Serving:

- Calories: 150
- Protein: 3g
- Carbohydrates: 15g
- Fat: 9g
- Fiber: 5g
- Sugar: 5g

Number of Servings:

- **4 servings**

Cooking Time:

- **30 minutes**

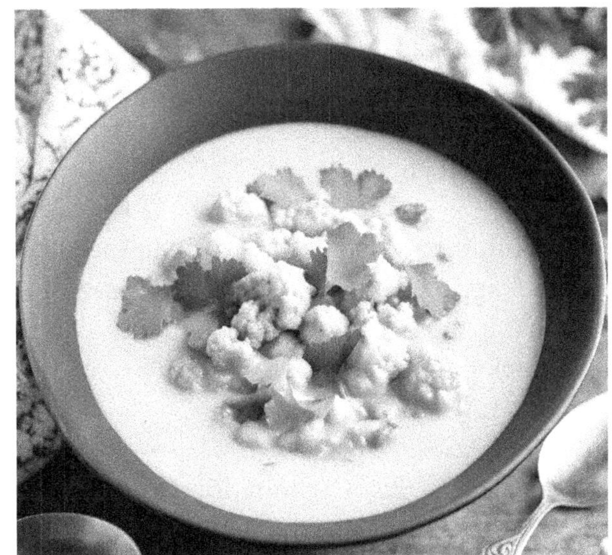

16. Roasted Turnips with Rosemary

Ingredients:

- 1 pound turnips, peeled and cut into wedges
- 2 tablespoons olive oil
- 2 teaspoons chopped fresh rosemary
- 1/4 teaspoon black pepper

Instructions:

1. Preheat the oven to 400°F (200°C) and line a baking sheet with parchment paper.
2. In a large bowl, toss the turnip wedges with olive oil, rosemary, and black pepper.
3. Spread the turnips in a single layer on the prepared baking sheet.
4. Roast for 25-30 minutes, stirring halfway through, until the turnips are tender and golden brown.
5. Serve immediately.

Nutrition Info per Serving:

- Calories: 100   Protein: 1g   Carbohydrates: 10g   Fat: 7g   Fiber: 3g   Sugar: 5g

Number of Servings:

- **4 servings**

Cooking Time:

- **30 minutes**

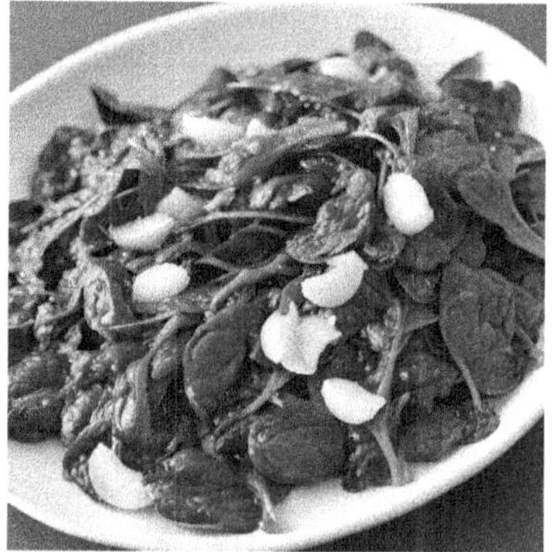

17. Sautéed Spinach and Garlic

Ingredients:

- 1 tablespoon olive oil
- 3 cloves garlic, minced
- 8 cups fresh spinach leaves
- 1/4 teaspoon black pepper
- 1 tablespoon lemon juice

Instructions:

1. Heat olive oil in a large skillet over medium heat. Add the garlic and cook for 1 minute until fragrant.
2. Add the spinach and cook, stirring frequently, until wilted, about 3-4 minutes.
3. Stir in the black pepper and lemon juice.
4. Serve immediately.

Nutrition Info per Serving:

- Calories: 70   Protein: 2g   Carbohydrates: 5g   Fat: 5g   Fiber: 2g Sugar: 1g

Number of Servings:

- **4 servings**

Cooking Time:

- **10 minutes**

18. Mashed Parsnips

Ingredients:

- 1 1/2 pounds parsnips, peeled and cut into chunks
- 2 tablespoons olive oil
- 1/4 cup low-fat milk
- 1/4 teaspoon black pepper
- 1/4 teaspoon nutmeg

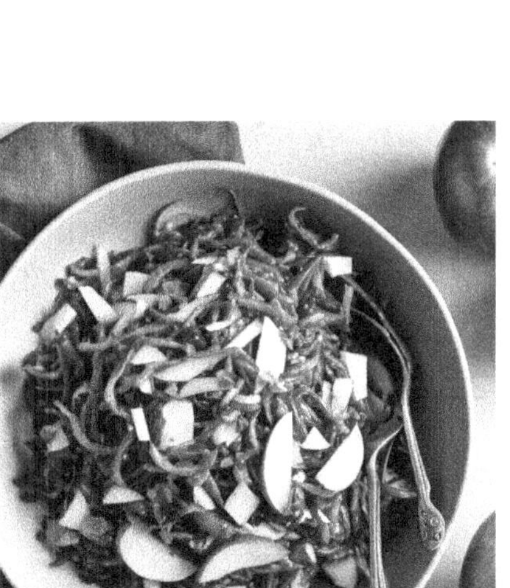

Instructions:

1. Bring a large pot of water to a boil. Add the parsnips and cook until tender, about 15-20 minutes.
2. Drain the parsnips and return them to the pot.
3. Add the olive oil, milk, black pepper, and nutmeg. Mash until smooth.
4. Serve immediately.

Nutrition Info per Serving:

- Calories: 150 Protein: 2g Carbohydrates: 20g Fat: 7g Fiber: 5g Sugar: 6g

Number of Servings:

- **4 servings**

Cooking Time:

- **20 minutes**

19. Red Cabbage Slaw with Apples

Ingredients:

- 4 cups shredded red cabbage
- 2 apples, thinly sliced
- 1/4 cup chopped walnuts
- 1/4 cup raisins
- 2 tablespoons apple cider vinegar
- 2 tablespoons olive oil
- 1 tablespoon honey
- 1/4 teaspoon black pepper

Instructions:

1. In a large bowl, combine the shredded red cabbage, sliced apples, chopped walnuts, and raisins.
2. In a small bowl, whisk together the apple cider vinegar, olive oil, honey, and black pepper.
3. Pour the dressing over the cabbage mixture and toss to coat.
4. Let the slaw sit for at least 15 minutes before serving to allow the flavors to meld.
5. Serve immediately.

Nutrition Info per Serving:

- Calories: 150 Protein: 2g Carbohydrates: 20g Fat: 8g Fiber: 4g Sugar: 12g

Number of Servings:

- **4 servings**

Cooking Time:

- **15 minutes**

20. Zucchini and Tomato Gratin

Ingredients:

- 2 large zucchinis, thinly sliced
- 3 large tomatoes, thinly sliced
- 1 large onion, thinly sliced
- 2 cloves garlic, minced
- 2 tablespoons olive oil
- 1/2 cup whole wheat breadcrumbs
- 1/4 cup grated Parmesan cheese
- 1 teaspoon dried oregano
- 1/4 teaspoon black pepper
- Fresh basil for garnish (optional)

Instructions:

1. Preheat the oven to 375°F (190°C).
2. In a large skillet, heat 1 tablespoon of olive oil over medium heat. Add the onion and garlic, and cook until softened, about 5 minutes.
3. In a large baking dish, layer half of the zucchini slices, followed by half of the tomato slices, and then half of the cooked onions and garlic. Repeat the layers.
4. In a small bowl, mix the breadcrumbs, Parmesan cheese, oregano, black pepper, and the remaining 1 tablespoon of olive oil.
5. Sprinkle the breadcrumb mixture evenly over the top of the layered vegetables.
6. Bake in the preheated oven for 25-30 minutes, until the top is golden brown and the vegetables are tender.
7. Garnish with fresh basil if desired and serve immediately.

Nutrition Info per Serving:

- Calories: 150
- Protein: 5g
- Carbohydrates: 15g
- Fat: 8g
- Fiber: 3g
- Sugar: 5g

Number of Servings:

- **4 servings**

Cooking Time:

- **30 minutes**

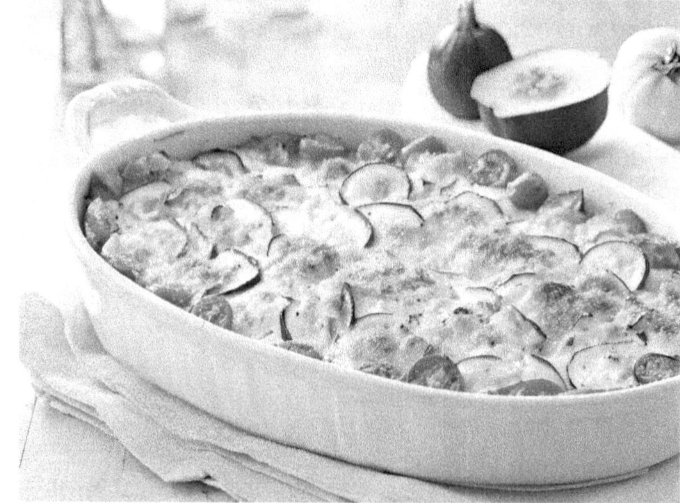

21. Miso Glazed Carrots

Ingredients:

- 1 pound carrots, peeled and cut into sticks
- 1 tablespoon olive oil
- 2 tablespoons white miso paste
- 1 tablespoon maple syrup
- 1 tablespoon rice vinegar
- 1 teaspoon grated fresh ginger
- 1/4 teaspoon black pepper
- 1 tablespoon sesame seeds (optional, for garnish)
- Fresh cilantro for garnish (optional)

Instructions:

1. Preheat the oven to 400°F (200°C) and line a baking sheet with parchment paper.
2. In a small bowl, whisk together the miso paste, maple syrup, rice vinegar, ginger, and black pepper.
3. In a large bowl, toss the carrot sticks with olive oil and the miso glaze until evenly coated.
4. Spread the carrots in a single layer on the prepared baking sheet.
5. Roast in the preheated oven for 20-25 minutes, stirring halfway through, until the carrots are tender and caramelized.
6. Sprinkle with sesame seeds and garnish with fresh cilantro if desired.
7. Serve immediately.

Nutrition Info per Serving:

- Calories: 120
- Protein: 2g
- Carbohydrates: 18g
- Fat: 5g
- Fiber: 3g
- Sugar: 10g

Number of Servings:

- **4 servings**

Cooking Time:

- **25 minutes**

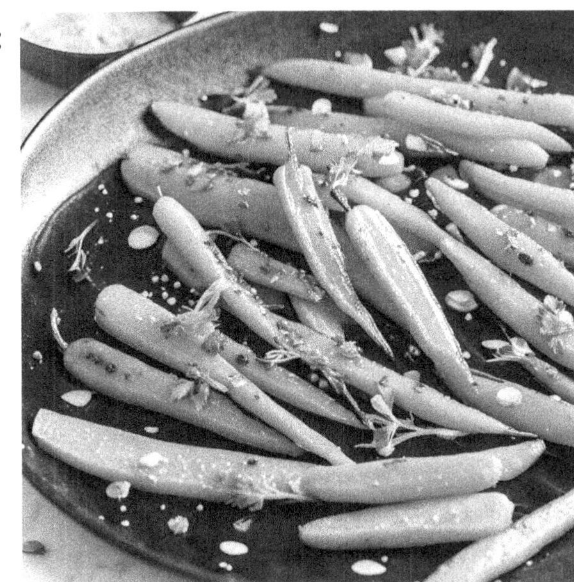

22. Tomato and Mozzarella Caprese

Ingredients:

- 4 large tomatoes, sliced
- 8 ounces fresh mozzarella, sliced
- 1/4 cup fresh basil leaves
- 2 tablespoons olive oil
- 1 tablespoon balsamic vinegar
- 1/4 teaspoon black pepper

Instructions:

1. On a large serving platter, arrange the tomato and mozzarella slices alternately in a circular pattern.
2. Tuck fresh basil leaves between the tomato and mozzarella slices.
3. Drizzle with olive oil and balsamic vinegar.
4. Sprinkle with black pepper.
5. Serve immediately.

Nutrition Info per Serving:

- Calories: 200
- Protein: 10g
- Carbohydrates: 6g
- Fat: 15g
- Fiber: 2g
- Sugar: 4g

Number of Servings:

- **4 servings**

Cooking Time:

- **10 minutes**

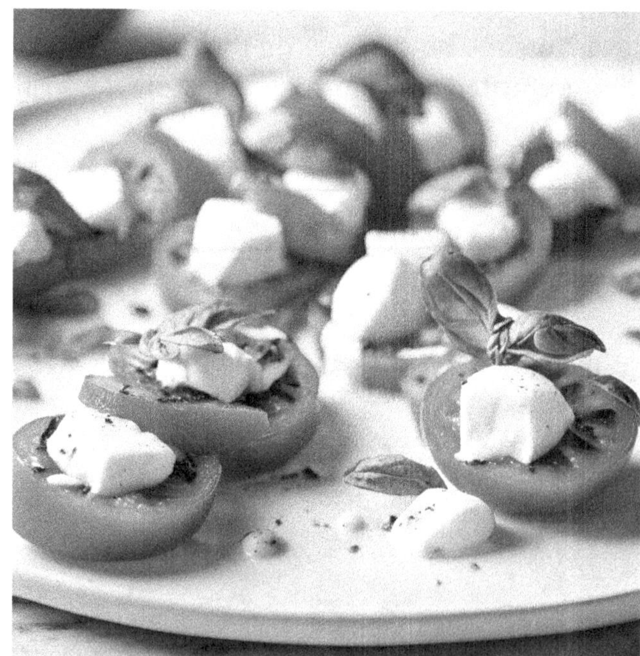

Fish and Seafood Recipes

1. Grilled Salmon with Dill Sauce

Ingredients:

- 4 salmon fillets (6 ounces each)
- 1 tablespoon olive oil
- 1/4 teaspoon black pepper
- 1/2 cup plain Greek yogurt
- 1 tablespoon fresh dill, chopped
- 1 tablespoon lemon juice
- 1 teaspoon Dijon mustard
- 1 garlic clove, minced

Instructions:

1. Preheat the grill to medium-high heat.
2. Brush the salmon fillets with olive oil and sprinkle with black pepper.
3. Grill the salmon for 4-5 minutes per side, until the fish is opaque and flakes easily with a fork.
4. In a small bowl, mix together the Greek yogurt, dill, lemon juice, Dijon mustard, and minced garlic to make the dill sauce.
5. Serve the grilled salmon with a dollop of dill sauce on top.

Nutrition Info per Serving:

- Calories: 300
- Protein: 34g
- Carbohydrates: 3g
- Fat: 18g
- Fiber: 0g
- Sugar: 1g

Number of Servings:

- **4 servings**

Cooking Time:

- **15 minutes**

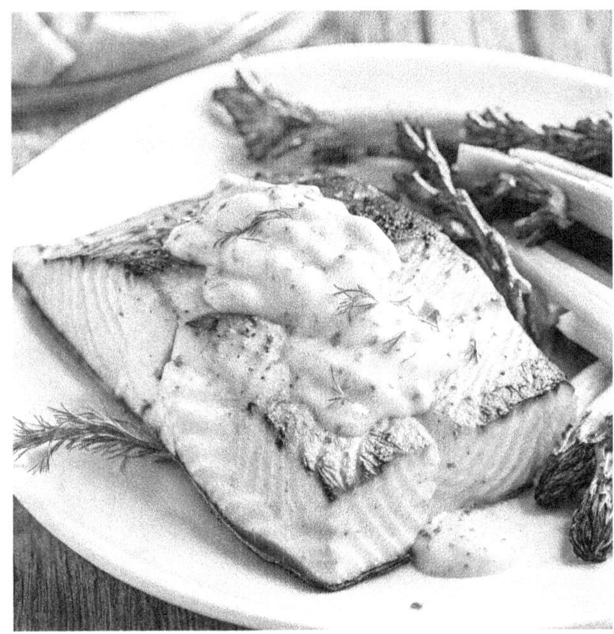

2. Baked Cod with Lemon and Capers

Ingredients:

- 4 cod fillets (6 ounces each)
- 2 tablespoons olive oil
- 1 lemon, thinly sliced
- 2 tablespoons capers, rinsed
- 1/4 teaspoon black pepper
- 2 cloves garlic, minced
- Fresh parsley for garnish (optional)

Instructions:

1. Preheat the oven to 400°F (200°C) and line a baking dish with parchment paper.
2. Place the cod fillets in the baking dish and drizzle with olive oil.
3. Sprinkle with black pepper and minced garlic.
4. Arrange the lemon slices and capers over the cod fillets.
5. Bake for 15-20 minutes, until the fish is opaque and flakes easily with a fork.
6. Garnish with fresh parsley if desired.
7. Serve immediately.

Nutrition Info per Serving:

- Calories: 220
- Protein: 35g
- Carbohydrates: 2g
- Fat: 8g
- Fiber: 0g
- Sugar: 0g

Number of Servings:

- **4 servings**

Cooking Time:

- **20 minutes**

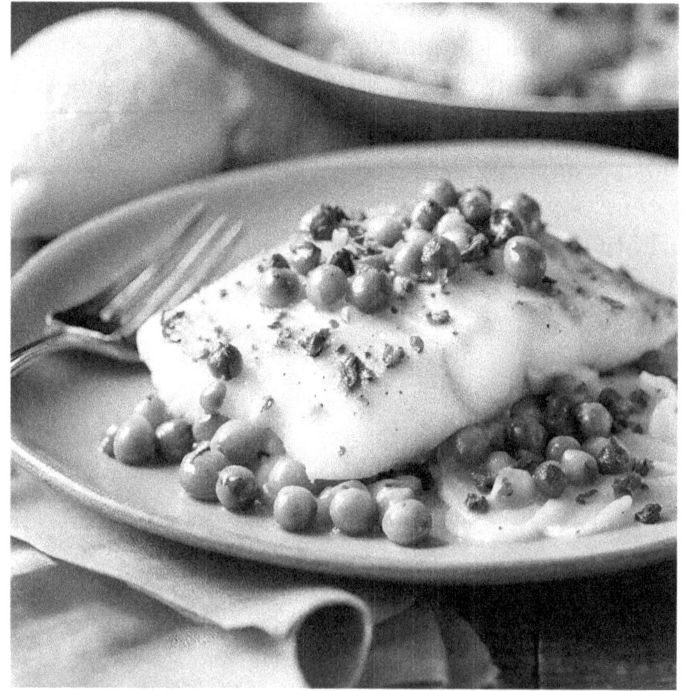

3. Shrimp Stir-Fry

Ingredients:

- 1 pound large shrimp, peeled and deveined
- 2 tablespoons olive oil
- 1 cup broccoli florets
- 1 cup sliced bell peppers (red, yellow, green)
- 1 cup snow peas
- 1/2 cup sliced carrots
- 1/2 cup sliced mushrooms
- 1/4 cup low-sodium soy sauce
- 2 tablespoons rice vinegar
- 1 tablespoon honey
- 1 teaspoon grated fresh ginger
- 1 garlic clove, minced

Instructions:

1. In a small bowl, whisk together the soy sauce, rice vinegar, honey, ginger, and garlic.
2. Heat 1 tablespoon of olive oil in a large skillet or wok over medium-high heat.
3. Add the shrimp and stir-fry until pink and cooked through, about 3-4 minutes. Remove shrimp from the skillet and set aside.
4. Add the remaining 1 tablespoon of olive oil to the skillet. Add the broccoli, bell peppers, snow peas, carrots, and mushrooms. Stir-fry until the vegetables are tender-crisp, about 5-7 minutes.
5. Return the shrimp to the skillet and pour the sauce over the top. Stir to coat and cook for an additional 2 minutes.
6. Serve immediately.

Nutrition Info per Serving:

- Calories: 250
- Protein: 25g
- Carbohydrates: 15g
- Fat: 10g
- Fiber: 3g
- Sugar: 6g

Number of Servings:

- **4 servings**

Cooking Time:

- **15 minutes**

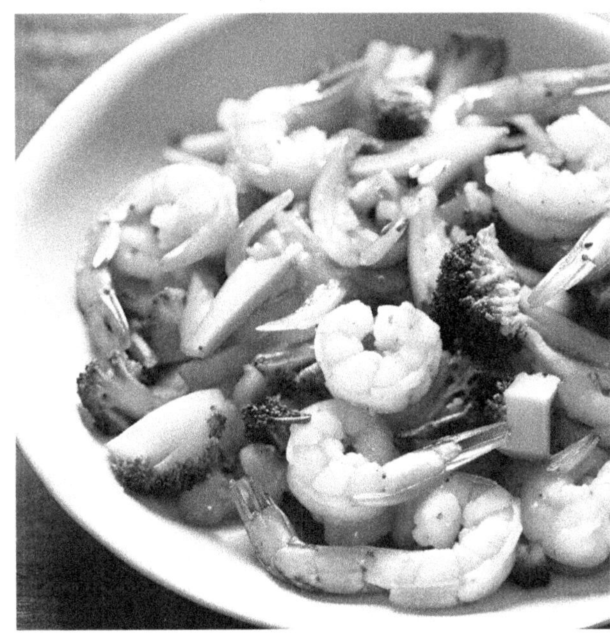

4. Sea Bass with Mango Salsa

Ingredients:

- 4 sea bass fillets (6 ounces each)
- 2 tablespoons olive oil
- 1/4 teaspoon black pepper
- 1 ripe mango, peeled and diced
- 1/4 cup red bell pepper, diced
- 1/4 cup red onion, finely diced
- 1 jalapeño, seeded and minced
- 1 tablespoon fresh lime juice
- 1 tablespoon fresh cilantro, chopped

Instructions:

1. Preheat the grill to medium-high heat.
2. Brush the sea bass fillets with olive oil and sprinkle with black pepper.
3. Grill the sea bass for 4-5 minutes per side, until the fish is opaque and flakes easily with a fork.
4. In a medium bowl, combine the mango, red bell pepper, red onion, jalapeño, lime juice, and cilantro to make the mango salsa.
5. Serve the grilled sea bass with mango salsa on top.

Nutrition Info per Serving:

- Calories: 300
- Protein: 30g
- Carbohydrates: 15g
- Fat: 15g
- Fiber: 2g
- Sugar: 12g

Number of Servings:

- **4 servings**

Cooking Time:

- **15 minutes**

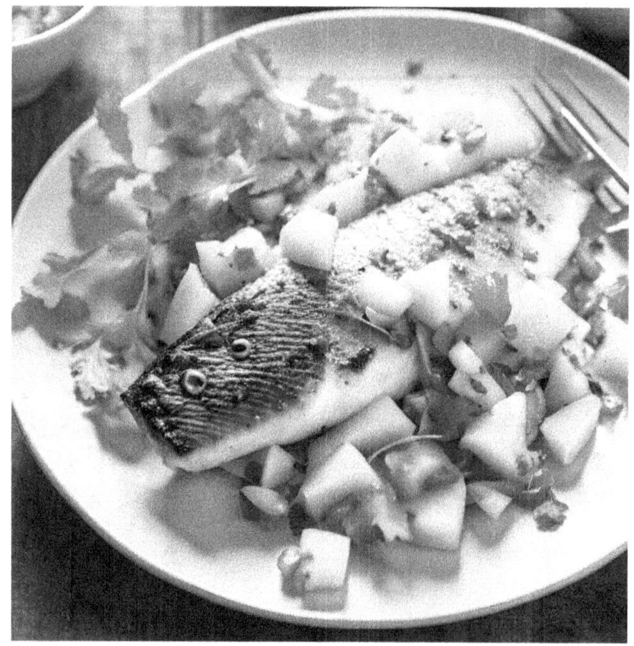

5. Tuna Steak with Olive Tapenade

Ingredients:

- 4 tuna steaks (6 ounces each)
- 2 tablespoons olive oil
- 1/4 teaspoon black pepper
- 1 cup pitted Kalamata olives
- 2 tablespoons capers, rinsed
- 2 cloves garlic, minced
- 1 tablespoon lemon juice
- 1 tablespoon fresh parsley, chopped

Instructions:

1. Preheat the grill to medium-high heat.
2. Brush the tuna steaks with 1 tablespoon of olive oil and sprinkle with black pepper.
3. Grill the tuna steaks for 3-4 minutes per side, until seared on the outside and slightly pink in the center.
4. In a food processor, combine the olives, capers, garlic, lemon juice, remaining 1 tablespoon olive oil, and parsley. Pulse until finely chopped and well mixed.
5. Serve the grilled tuna steaks with a generous spoonful of olive tapenade on top.

Nutrition Info per Serving:

- Calories: 300
- Protein: 35g
- Carbohydrates: 3g
- Fat: 18g
- Fiber: 2g
- Sugar: 0g

Number of Servings:

- **4 servings**

Cooking Time:

- **15 minutes**

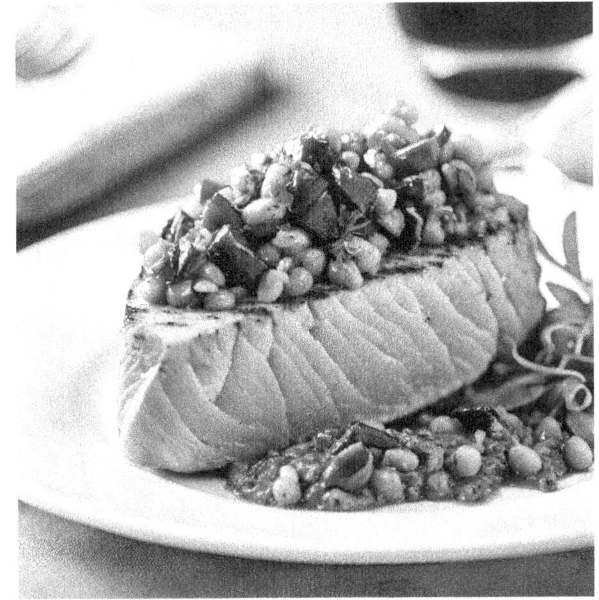

6. Crab Cakes with Yogurt Dipping Sauce

Ingredients:

- 1 pound lump crab meat
- 1/2 cup whole wheat breadcrumbs
- 1/4 cup diced red bell pepper
- 1/4 cup diced green onion
- 1/4 cup plain Greek yogurt
- 1 egg, beaten
- 1 tablespoon Dijon mustard
- 1 tablespoon lemon juice
- 1/4 teaspoon black pepper
- 2 tablespoons olive oil (for frying)

Yogurt Dipping Sauce:

- 1/2 cup plain Greek yogurt
- 1 tablespoon lemon juice
- 1 tablespoon fresh dill, chopped
- 1 garlic clove, minced

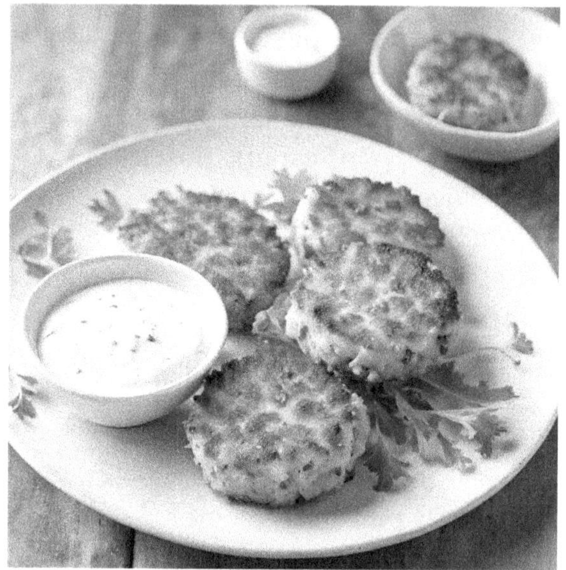

Instructions:

1. In a large bowl, combine the crab meat, breadcrumbs, red bell pepper, green onion, Greek yogurt, egg, Dijon mustard, lemon juice, and black pepper. Mix until well combined.
2. Form the mixture into 8 patties.
3. Heat the olive oil in a large skillet over medium heat. Fry the crab cakes for 3-4 minutes per side, until golden brown and cooked through.
4. In a small bowl, whisk together the yogurt, lemon juice, dill, and minced garlic to make the dipping sauce.
5. Serve the crab cakes warm with the yogurt dipping sauce.

Nutrition Info per Serving:

- Calories: 250
- Protein: 25g
- Carbohydrates: 10g
- Fat: 12g
- Fiber: 2g
- Sugar: 2g

Number of Servings:

- **4 servings (2 crab cakes each)**

Cooking Time:

- **20 minutes**

7. Baked Trout with Almonds

Ingredients:

- 4 trout fillets (6 ounces each)
- 2 tablespoons olive oil
- 1/4 cup sliced almonds
- 2 cloves garlic, minced
- 1 tablespoon lemon juice
- 1 tablespoon fresh parsley, chopped
- 1/4 teaspoon black pepper

Instructions:

1. Preheat the oven to 375°F (190°C) and line a baking sheet with parchment paper.
2. Place the trout fillets on the prepared baking sheet and drizzle with olive oil and lemon juice. Sprinkle with black pepper.
3. In a small bowl, mix the sliced almonds, minced garlic, and chopped parsley.
4. Sprinkle the almond mixture evenly over the trout fillets.
5. Bake for 15-20 minutes, until the trout is opaque and flakes easily with a fork.
6. Serve immediately.

Nutrition Info per Serving:

- Calories: 300
- Protein: 30g
- Carbohydrates: 3g
- Fat: 18g
- Fiber: 2g
- Sugar: 1g

Number of Servings:

- **4 servings**

Cooking Time:

- **20 minutes**

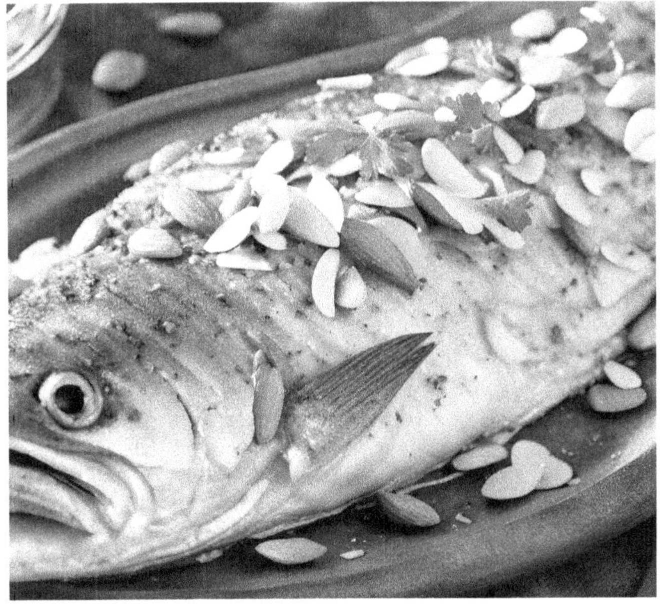

8. Grilled Mahi Mahi with Pineapple Salsa
Ingredients:

- 4 mahi mahi fillets (6 ounces each)
- 2 tablespoons olive oil
- 1/4 teaspoon black pepper

Pineapple Salsa:

- 1 cup fresh pineapple, diced
- 1/4 cup red bell pepper, diced
- 1/4 cup red onion, finely diced
- 1 jalapeño, seeded and minced
- 1 tablespoon fresh lime juice
- 1 tablespoon fresh cilantro, chopped

Instructions:

1. Preheat the grill to medium-high heat.
2. Brush the mahi mahi fillets with olive oil and sprinkle with black pepper.
3. Grill the mahi mahi for 4-5 minutes per side, until the fish is opaque and flakes easily with a fork.
4. In a medium bowl, combine the pineapple, red bell pepper, red onion, jalapeño, lime juice, and cilantro to make the pineapple salsa.
5. Serve the grilled mahi mahi with pineapple salsa on top.

Nutrition Info per Serving:

- Calories: 250
- Protein: 30g
- Carbohydrates: 10g
- Fat: 10g
- Fiber: 2g
- Sugar: 8g

Number of Servings:

- **4 servings**

Cooking Time:

- **15 minutes**

9. Seared Scallops with Pea Puree

Ingredients:

- 1 pound large sea scallops
- 2 tablespoons olive oil
- 1/4 teaspoon black pepper
- 2 cups frozen peas
- 1/2 cup low-sodium vegetable broth
- 1 garlic clove, minced
- 1 tablespoon lemon juice
- 1 tablespoon fresh mint, chopped (optional, for garnish)

Instructions:

1. In a medium saucepan, bring the vegetable broth to a boil. Add the frozen peas and cook for 3-5 minutes until tender.
2. Drain the peas and transfer them to a blender. Add the minced garlic and lemon juice, and blend until smooth. Set aside.
3. Pat the scallops dry with a paper towel and sprinkle with black pepper.
4. Heat olive oil in a large skillet over medium-high heat. Add the scallops and sear for 2-3 minutes per side, until they are golden brown and opaque in the center.
5. Serve the seared scallops on a bed of pea puree. Garnish with fresh mint if desired.

Nutrition Info per Serving:

- Calories: 300
- Protein: 28g
- Carbohydrates: 15g
- Fat: 12g
- Fiber: 5g
- Sugar: 4g

Number of Servings:

- **4 servings**

Cooking Time:

- **15 minutes**

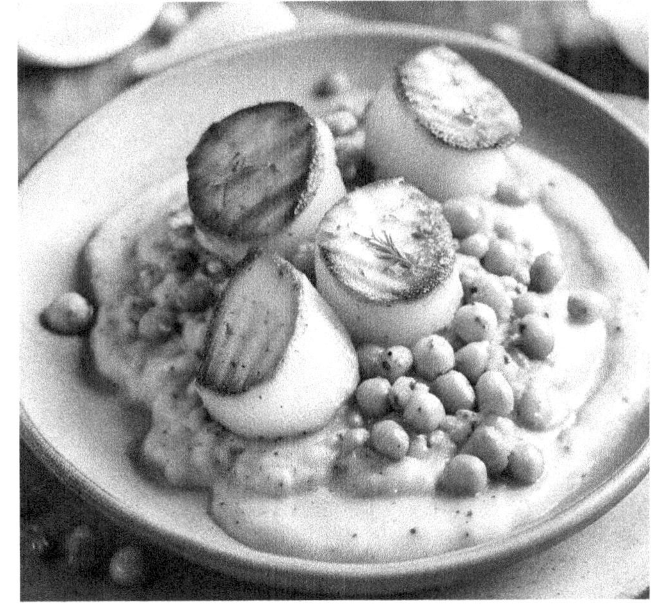

10. Fish Tacos with Cabbage Slaw

Ingredients:

- 1 pound white fish fillets (such as cod or tilapia)
- 2 tablespoons olive oil
- 1/4 teaspoon black pepper
- 8 small corn tortillas
- 1/2 cup plain Greek yogurt
- 1 tablespoon lime juice
- 1 cup shredded cabbage
- 1/4 cup chopped cilantro
- 1 jalapeño, seeded and minced
- 1 avocado, sliced

Instructions:

1. Preheat the grill to medium-high heat.
2. Brush the fish fillets with olive oil and sprinkle with black pepper.
3. Grill the fish for 3-4 minutes per side, until opaque and flaky. Remove from heat and set aside.
4. In a small bowl, mix the Greek yogurt and lime juice to make the sauce.
5. In a medium bowl, combine the shredded cabbage, chopped cilantro, and minced jalapeño to make the slaw.
6. Warm the corn tortillas on the grill or in a skillet.
7. Assemble the tacos by placing pieces of grilled fish in each tortilla. Top with cabbage slaw, a drizzle of yogurt sauce, and avocado slices.
8. Serve immediately.

Nutrition Info per Serving:

- Calories: 300
- Protein: 20g
- Carbohydrates: 25g
- Fat: 12g
- Fiber: 6g
- Sugar: 3g

Number of Servings:

- 4 servings (2 tacos each)

Cooking Time:

- 20 minutes

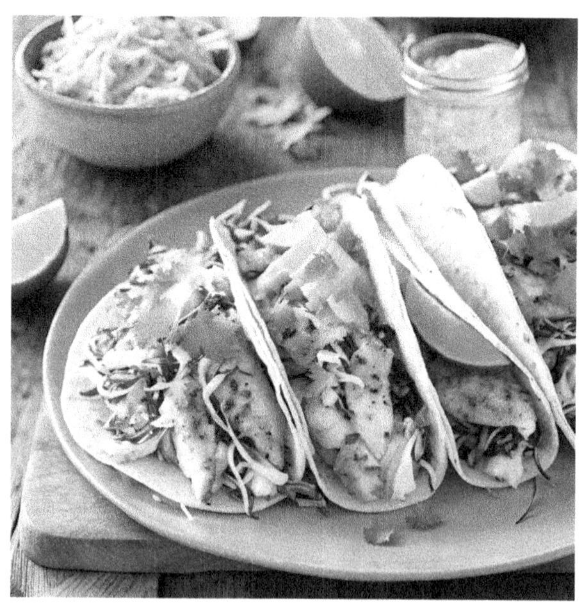

11. Sardines on Toast

Ingredients:

- 1 can (4 ounces) sardines in olive oil, drained
- 4 slices whole grain bread, toasted
- 1 tablespoon lemon juice
- 1 garlic clove, minced
- 1/4 teaspoon black pepper
- 1 tablespoon fresh parsley, chopped (optional)

Instructions:

1. In a small bowl, mash the sardines with a fork. Add the lemon juice, minced garlic, and black pepper. Mix well.
2. Spread the sardine mixture evenly over the toasted bread slices.
3. Garnish with fresh parsley if desired.
4. Serve immediately.

Nutrition Info per Serving:

- Calories: 200
- Protein: 12g
- Carbohydrates: 20g
- Fat: 8g
- Fiber: 3g
- Sugar: 2g

Number of Servings:

- **4 servings**

Cooking Time:

- **10 minutes**

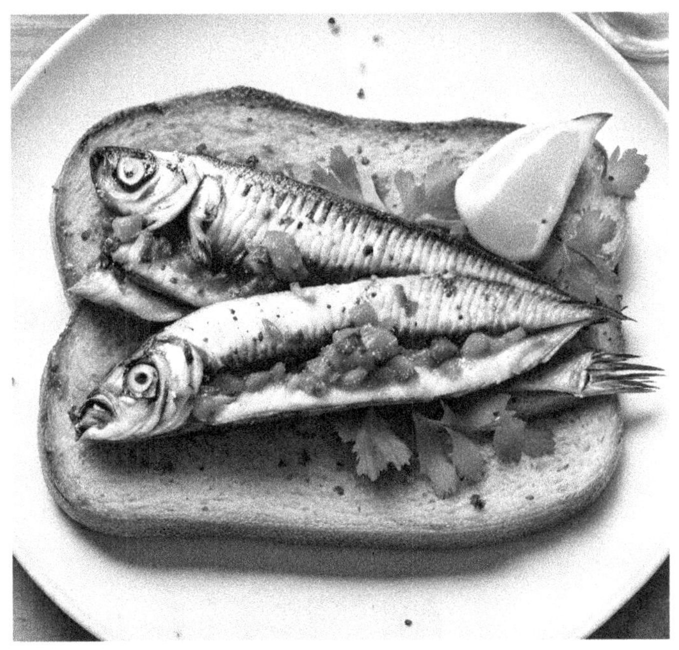

12. Halibut with Herb Butter

Ingredients:

- 4 halibut fillets (6 ounces each)
- 2 tablespoons olive oil
- 1/4 teaspoon black pepper
- 2 tablespoons unsalted butter, softened
- 1 tablespoon fresh parsley, chopped
- 1 tablespoon fresh dill, chopped
- 1 tablespoon lemon juice
- Lemon wedges for serving (optional)

Instructions:

1. Preheat the oven to 400°F (200°C) and line a baking sheet with parchment paper.
2. Brush the halibut fillets with olive oil and sprinkle with black pepper.
3. In a small bowl, mix the softened butter, chopped parsley, dill, and lemon juice.
4. Place the halibut fillets on the prepared baking sheet and spread the herb butter mixture over the top of each fillet.
5. Bake for 15-20 minutes, until the fish is opaque and flakes easily with a fork.
6. Serve with lemon wedges if desired.

Nutrition Info per Serving:

- Calories: 300
- Protein: 32g
- Carbohydrates: 1g
- Fat: 18g
- Fiber: 0g
- Sugar: 0g

Number of Servings:

- **4 servings**

Cooking Time:

- **20 minutes**

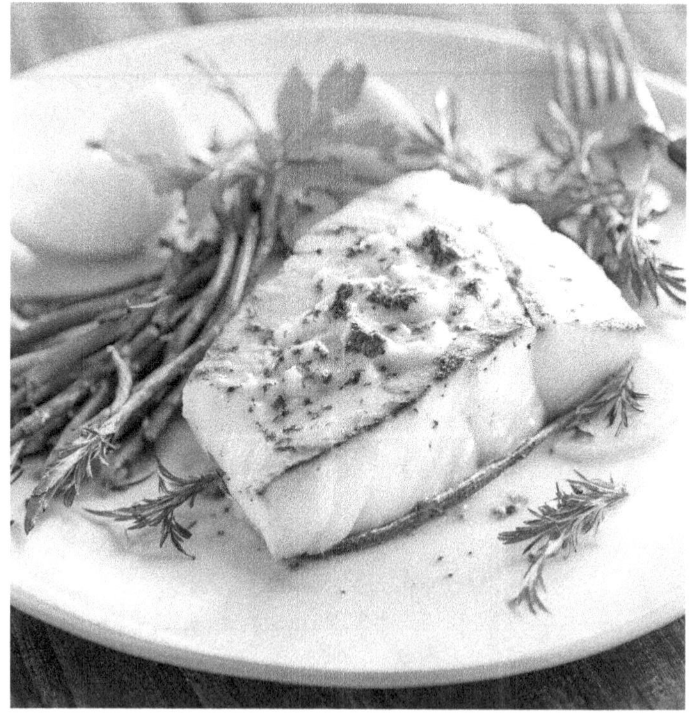

13. Poached Salmon with Cucumber Dill Salad

Ingredients:
- 4 salmon fillets (6 ounces each)
- 4 cups low-sodium vegetable broth
- 1 lemon, sliced
- 1 tablespoon fresh dill, chopped
- 2 cucumbers, thinly sliced
- 1/4 cup plain Greek yogurt
- 1 tablespoon lemon juice
- 1 tablespoon fresh dill, chopped

Instructions:
1. In a large skillet, bring the vegetable broth and lemon slices to a simmer.
2. Add the salmon fillets to the skillet and poach for 10-12 minutes, until the salmon is opaque and flakes easily with a fork.
3. While the salmon is poaching, combine the cucumbers, Greek yogurt, lemon juice, and dill in a medium bowl to make the cucumber dill salad.
4. Serve the poached salmon with the cucumber dill salad on the side.

Nutrition Info per Serving:
- Calories: 300
- Protein: 34g
- Carbohydrates: 8g
- Fat: 16g
- Fiber: 2g
- Sugar: 4g

Number of Servings:
- **4 servings**

Cooking Time:
- **15 minutes**

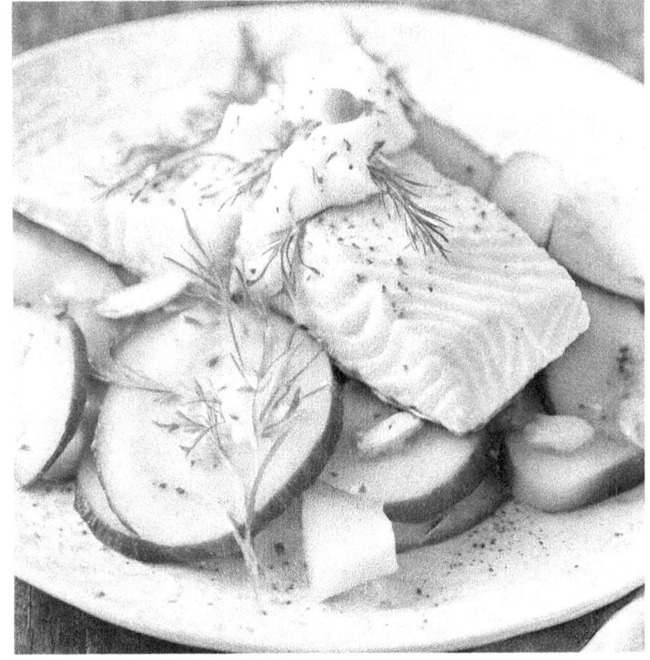

14. Haddock in Parchment with Vegetables

Ingredients:

- 4 haddock fillets (6 ounces each)
- 2 tablespoons olive oil
- 2 zucchini, thinly sliced
- 2 carrots, thinly sliced
- 1 red bell pepper, thinly sliced
- 1 lemon, thinly sliced
- 1 teaspoon dried thyme
- 1/4 teaspoon black pepper

Instructions:

1. Preheat the oven to 375°F (190°C).
2. Cut 4 large pieces of parchment paper and place a haddock fillet in the center of each.
3. Arrange the zucchini, carrots, and bell pepper slices around each fillet. Drizzle with olive oil and sprinkle with thyme and black pepper.
4. Top each fillet with lemon slices.
5. Fold the parchment paper over the fish and vegetables, crimping the edges to seal the packets.
6. Place the packets on a baking sheet and bake for 20-25 minutes, until the fish is opaque and flakes easily with a fork.
7. Serve immediately.

Nutrition Info per Serving:

- Calories: 280
- Protein: 32g
- Carbohydrates: 12g
- Fat: 12g
- Fiber: 4g
- Sugar: 6g

Number of Servings:

- **4 servings**

Cooking Time:

- **25 minutes**

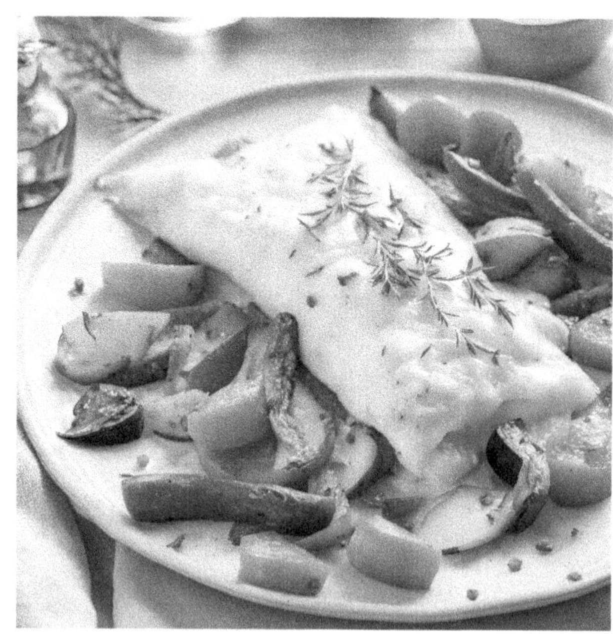

15. Shrimp and Asparagus Risotto

Ingredients:

- 1 pound large shrimp, peeled and deveined
- 1 bunch asparagus, trimmed and cut into 1-inch pieces
- 1 cup Arborio rice
- 4 cups low-sodium vegetable broth
- 1/2 cup white wine (optional)
- 1 onion, finely diced
- 2 cloves garlic, minced
- 2 tablespoons olive oil
- 1/4 cup grated Parmesan cheese (optional)
- 1/4 teaspoon black pepper

Instructions:

1. Heat the vegetable broth in a saucepan and keep it warm over low heat.
2. In a large skillet, heat 1 tablespoon of olive oil over medium heat. Add the onion and garlic, and cook until softened, about 5 minutes.
3. Add the Arborio rice and cook, stirring frequently, for 2 minutes.
4. Pour in the white wine (if using) and cook until it is mostly absorbed.
5. Begin adding the warm broth, one ladle at a time, stirring constantly and waiting until the liquid is absorbed before adding more. Continue until the rice is creamy and cooked through, about 20 minutes.
6. Meanwhile, in a separate skillet, heat the remaining 1 tablespoon of olive oil over medium heat. Add the shrimp and asparagus, and cook until the shrimp are pink and the asparagus is tender, about 5-7 minutes.
7. Stir the shrimp and asparagus into the risotto. Add the Parmesan cheese (if using) and black pepper.
8. Serve immediately.

Nutrition Info per Serving:

- Calories: 350
- Protein: 28g
- Carbohydrates: 45g
- Fat: 10g
- Fiber: 3g
- Sugar: 4g

Number of Servings:

- **4 servings**

Cooking Time:

- **30 minutes**

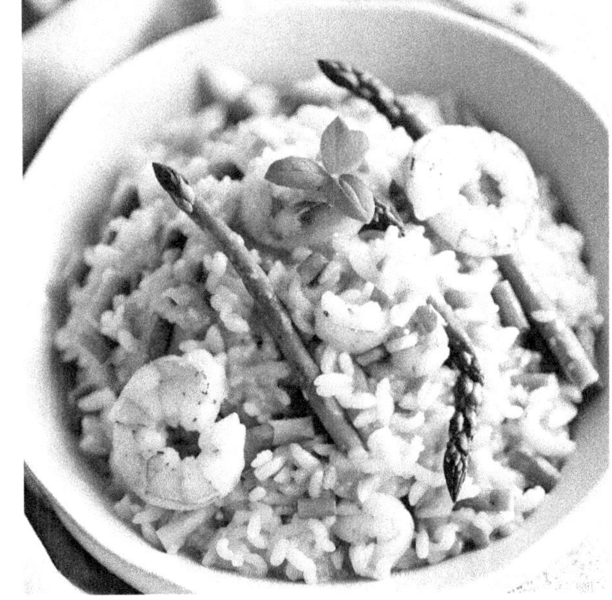

16. Fish Soup with Tomatoes

Ingredients:

- 1 pound white fish fillets (such as cod or tilapia), cut into bite-sized pieces
- 1 can (14.5 ounces) diced tomatoes
- 4 cups low-sodium vegetable broth
- 1 onion, diced
- 2 cloves garlic, minced
- 1 carrot, sliced
- 1 celery stalk, sliced
- 2 tablespoons olive oil
- 1 teaspoon dried thyme
- 1/4 teaspoon black pepper
- Fresh parsley for garnish (optional)

Instructions:

1. Heat olive oil in a large pot over medium heat. Add the onion, garlic, carrot, and celery. Cook until softened, about 5 minutes.
2. Add the diced tomatoes, vegetable broth, thyme, and black pepper. Bring to a boil, then reduce heat and simmer for 10 minutes.
3. Add the fish pieces to the pot and simmer for another 5-7 minutes, until the fish is opaque and flakes easily with a fork.
4. Garnish with fresh parsley if desired.
5. Serve immediately.

Nutrition Info per Serving:

- Calories: 220
- Protein: 30g
- Carbohydrates: 12g
- Fat: 8g
- Fiber: 3g
- Sugar: 5g

Number of Servings:

- **4 servings**

Cooking Time:

- **20 minutes**

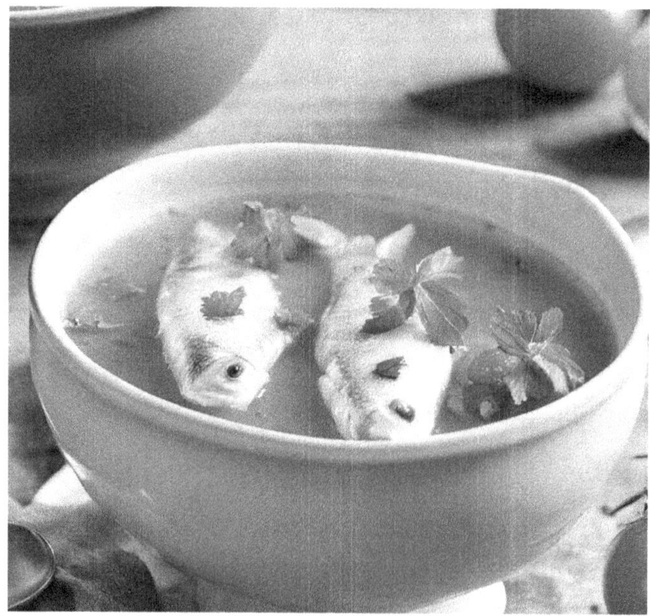

17. Scallop Ceviche

Ingredients:

- 1 pound sea scallops, cut into small pieces
- 1/2 cup fresh lime juice
- 1/4 cup fresh lemon juice
- 1/2 red onion, finely diced
- 1 jalapeño, seeded and minced
- 1/2 cup diced tomato
- 1/4 cup chopped cilantro
- 1 avocado, diced
- 1/4 teaspoon black pepper

Instructions:

1. In a large bowl, combine the scallops, lime juice, lemon juice, red onion, and jalapeño. Mix well.
2. Cover and refrigerate for 2-3 hours, until the scallops are opaque and firm.
3. Stir in the diced tomato, cilantro, and black pepper.
4. Just before serving, gently fold in the diced avocado.
5. Serve immediately.

Nutrition Info per Serving:

- Calories: 200
- Protein: 20g
- Carbohydrates: 12g
- Fat: 8g
- Fiber: 4g
- Sugar: 3g

Number of Servings:

- **4 servings**

Cooking Time:

- **15 minutes (plus 2-3 hours chilling time)**

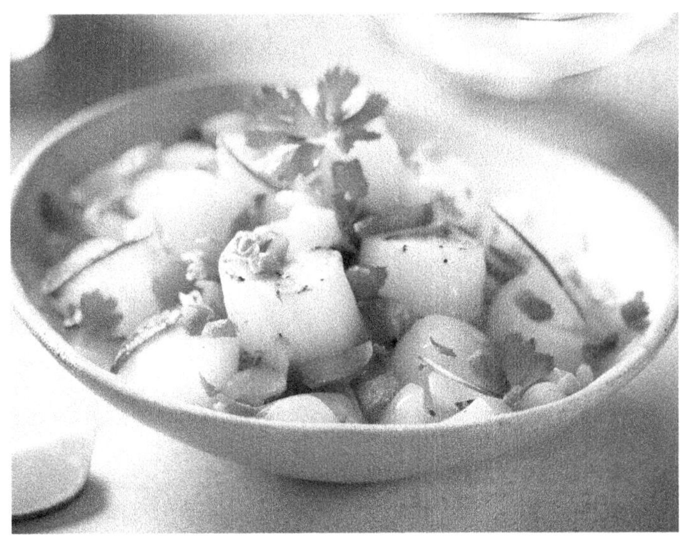

18. Monkfish Stew

Ingredients:

- 1 pound monkfish fillets, cut into bite-sized pieces
- 2 tablespoons olive oil
- 1 large onion, diced
- 2 cloves garlic, minced
- 1 can (14.5 ounces) diced tomatoes
- 4 cups low-sodium vegetable broth
- 2 carrots, sliced
- 2 celery stalks, sliced
- 1 teaspoon dried thyme
- 1 teaspoon smoked paprika
- 1/4 teaspoon black pepper
- Fresh parsley for garnish (optional)

Instructions:

1. Heat olive oil in a large pot over medium heat. Add the onion and garlic, and cook until softened, about 5 minutes.
2. Add the carrots and celery, and cook for another 5 minutes.
3. Stir in the diced tomatoes, vegetable broth, thyme, smoked paprika, and black pepper. Bring to a boil, then reduce heat and simmer for 15 minutes.
4. Add the monkfish pieces and simmer for an additional 10 minutes, until the fish is opaque and cooked through.
5. Garnish with fresh parsley if desired.
6. Serve immediately.

Nutrition Info per Serving:

- Calories: 250
- Protein: 25g
- Carbohydrates: 15g
- Fat: 10g
- Fiber: 4g
- Sugar: 7g

Number of Servings:

- **4 servings**

Cooking Time:

- **30 minutes**

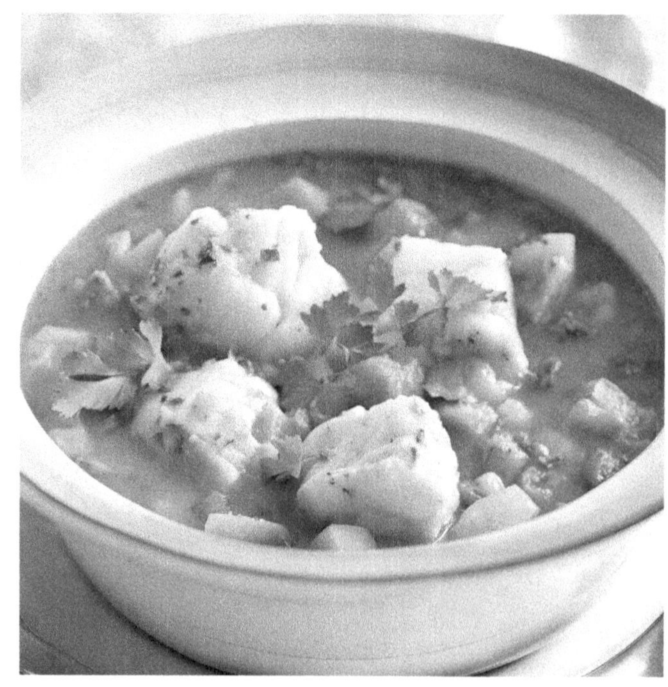

19. Catfish with Black Bean Sauce

Ingredients:

- 4 catfish fillets (6 ounces each)
- 2 tablespoons olive oil
- 1/4 teaspoon black pepper
- 1/2 cup canned black beans, rinsed and drained
- 1/4 cup low-sodium soy sauce
- 1 tablespoon rice vinegar
- 1 tablespoon honey
- 1 garlic clove, minced
- 1 teaspoon grated fresh ginger
- 2 green onions, sliced

Instructions:

1. Preheat the oven to 375°F (190°C).
2. Brush the catfish fillets with 1 tablespoon of olive oil and sprinkle with black pepper. Place on a baking sheet lined with parchment paper.
3. Bake for 15-20 minutes, until the fish is opaque and flakes easily with a fork.
4. Meanwhile, in a small saucepan, heat the remaining 1 tablespoon of olive oil over medium heat. Add the garlic and ginger, and cook for 1 minute until fragrant.
5. Stir in the black beans, soy sauce, rice vinegar, and honey. Simmer for 5 minutes.
6. Pour the black bean sauce over the baked catfish fillets and garnish with sliced green onions.
7. Serve immediately.

Nutrition Info per Serving:

- Calories: 300
- Protein: 28g
- Carbohydrates: 12g
- Fat: 14g
- Fiber: 2g
- Sugar: 4g

Number of Servings:

- **4 servings**

Cooking Time:

- **25 minutes**

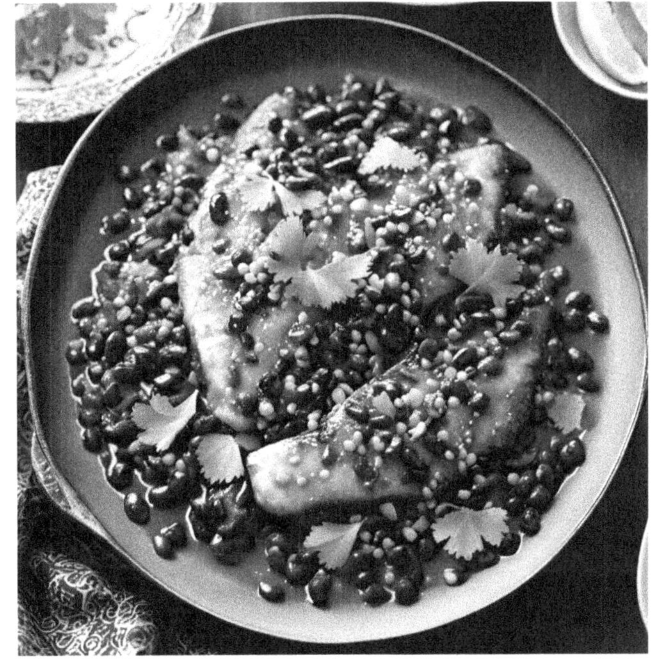

20. Tilapia with Tomato Basil Sauce

Ingredients:

- 4 tilapia fillets (6 ounces each)
- 2 tablespoons olive oil
- 1/4 teaspoon black pepper
- 1 large onion, diced
- 2 cloves garlic, minced
- 4 tomatoes, chopped
- 1/4 cup fresh basil, chopped
- 1 tablespoon lemon juice
- Fresh basil for garnish (optional)

Instructions:

1. Preheat the oven to 375°F (190°C).
2. Brush the tilapia fillets with 1 tablespoon of olive oil and sprinkle with black pepper. Place on a baking sheet lined with parchment paper.
3. Bake for 15-20 minutes, until the fish is opaque and flakes easily with a fork.
4. Meanwhile, in a large skillet, heat the remaining 1 tablespoon of olive oil over medium heat. Add the onion and garlic, and cook until softened, about 5 minutes.
5. Add the chopped tomatoes and cook for another 5 minutes until they begin to break down.
6. Stir in the fresh basil and lemon juice, and cook for an additional 2 minutes.
7. Serve the tilapia topped with the tomato basil sauce. Garnish with additional fresh basil if desired.

Nutrition Info per Serving:

- Calories: 250
- Protein: 30g
- Carbohydrates: 10g
- Fat: 10g
- Fiber: 2g
- Sugar: 5g

Number of Servings:

- **4 servings**

Cooking Time:

- **25 minutes**

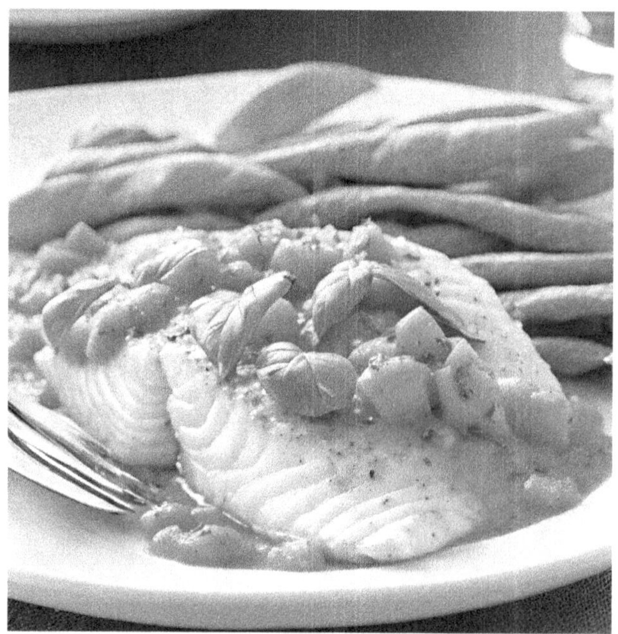

21. Crab Stuffed Flounder

Ingredients:

- 4 flounder fillets (6 ounces each)
- 1 cup lump crab meat
- 1/2 cup whole wheat breadcrumbs
- 1/4 cup plain Greek yogurt
- 1 egg, beaten
- 1 tablespoon Dijon mustard
- 1 tablespoon lemon juice
- 1 garlic clove, minced
- 1/4 teaspoon black pepper
- 1 tablespoon olive oil
- Fresh parsley for garnish (optional)

Instructions:

1. Preheat the oven to 375°F (190°C).
2. In a medium bowl, combine the crab meat, breadcrumbs, Greek yogurt, beaten egg, Dijon mustard, lemon juice, minced garlic, and black pepper.
3. Spread the crab mixture evenly over each flounder fillet and roll up, securing with toothpicks if necessary.
4. Place the stuffed flounder fillets in a baking dish and drizzle with olive oil.
5. Bake for 20-25 minutes, until the fish is opaque and cooked through.
6. Garnish with fresh parsley if desired.
7. Serve immediately.

Nutrition Info per Serving:

- Calories: 300
- Protein: 32g
- Carbohydrates: 10g
- Fat: 14g
- Fiber: 2g
- Sugar: 1g

Number of Servings:

- **4 servings**

Cooking Time:

- **25 minutes**

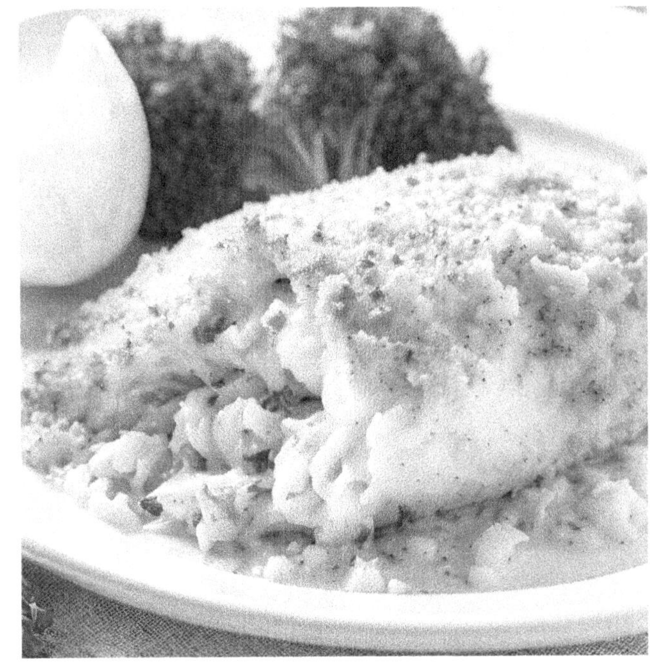

22. Seared Tuna with Sesame Seeds

Ingredients:

- 4 tuna steaks (6 ounces each)
- 2 tablespoons sesame oil
- 1/4 cup sesame seeds
- 1/4 teaspoon black pepper
- 1 tablespoon soy sauce
- 1 tablespoon rice vinegar
- 1 teaspoon honey
- 1 teaspoon grated fresh ginger
- 1 green onion, sliced

Instructions:

1. Pat the tuna steaks dry and sprinkle with black pepper.
2. Spread the sesame seeds on a plate and press each tuna steak into the seeds, coating both sides.
3. Heat the sesame oil in a large skillet over medium-high heat.
4. Sear the tuna steaks for 1-2 minutes per side, until the sesame seeds are golden brown and the tuna is cooked to your desired level of doneness.
5. In a small bowl, whisk together the soy sauce, rice vinegar, honey, and grated ginger to make the sauce.
6. Serve the seared tuna with the sauce drizzled on top and garnish with sliced green onion.
7. Serve immediately.

Nutrition Info per Serving:

- Calories: 350
- Protein: 38g
- Carbohydrates: 6g
- Fat: 18g
- Fiber: 2g
- Sugar: 2g

Number of Servings:

- **4 servings**

Cooking Time:

- **10 minutes**

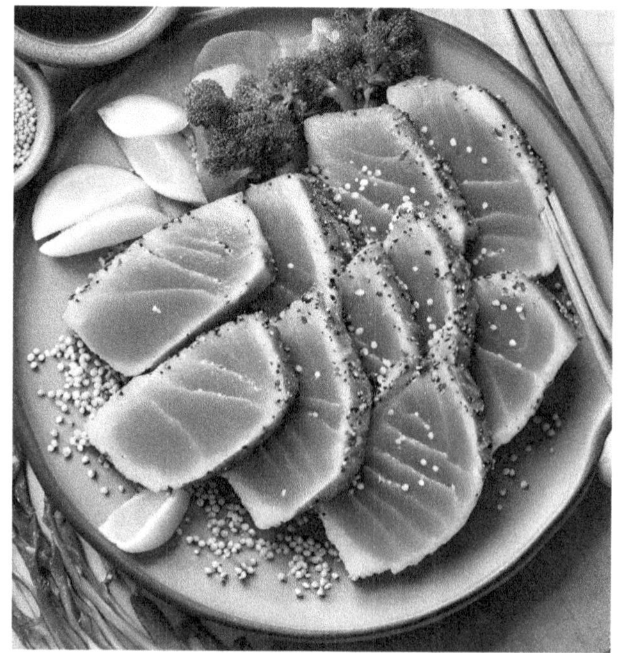

23. Fish Curry with Coconut Milk

Ingredients:

- 1 pound white fish fillets (such as cod or tilapia), cut into bite-sized pieces
- 2 tablespoons olive oil
- 1 large onion, diced
- 2 cloves garlic, minced
- 1 tablespoon grated fresh ginger
- 2 tablespoons curry powder
- 1 teaspoon ground turmeric
- 1/4 teaspoon black pepper
- 1 can (14 ounces) coconut milk
- 1 cup low-sodium vegetable broth
- 1 cup diced tomatoes
- 1 cup green beans, trimmed and cut into 1-inch pieces
- Fresh cilantro for garnish (optional)

Instructions:

1. Heat the olive oil in a large pot over medium heat. Add the onion, garlic, and ginger, and cook until softened, about 5 minutes.
2. Add the curry powder, turmeric, and black pepper, and cook for another minute until fragrant.
3. Stir in the coconut milk, vegetable broth, and diced tomatoes. Bring to a simmer.
4. Add the fish pieces and green beans. Cook for 10-15 minutes, until the fish is opaque and cooked through and the green beans are tender.
5. Garnish with fresh cilantro if desired.
6. Serve immediately.

Nutrition Info per Serving:

- Calories: 350
- Protein: 30g
- Carbohydrates: 12g
- Fat: 20g
- Fiber: 4g
- Sugar: 5g

Number of Servings:

- **4 servings**

Cooking Time:

- **25 minutes**

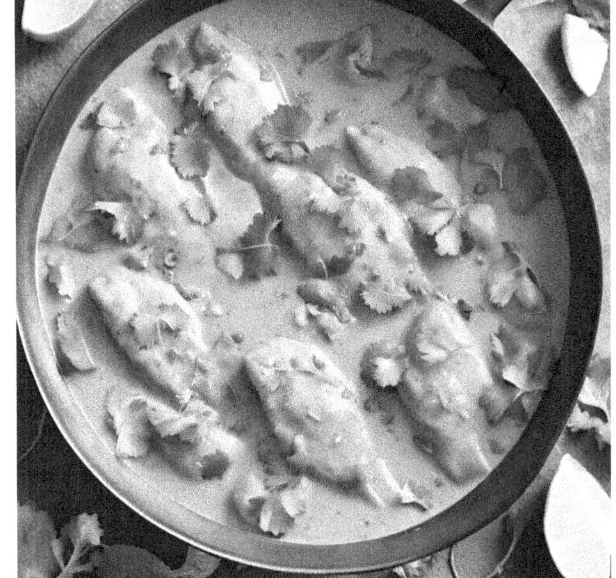

24. Anchovy Pasta

Ingredients:

- 8 ounces whole wheat spaghetti
- 2 tablespoons olive oil
- 1 can (2 ounces) anchovy fillets, drained and chopped
- 2 cloves garlic, minced
- 1/4 teaspoon black pepper
- 1/4 teaspoon red pepper flakes
- 1/4 cup chopped fresh parsley
- 1 tablespoon lemon juice
- 1/4 cup grated Parmesan cheese (optional)

Instructions:

1. Cook the spaghetti according to package instructions. Drain and set aside.
2. In a large skillet, heat the olive oil over medium heat. Add the garlic, anchovy fillets, black pepper, and red pepper flakes. Cook for 2-3 minutes, until the garlic is fragrant and the anchovies have dissolved.
3. Add the cooked spaghetti to the skillet and toss to coat in the anchovy mixture.
4. Stir in the parsley and lemon juice.
5. Serve immediately, topped with grated Parmesan cheese if desired.

Nutrition Info per Serving:

- Calories: 400
- Protein: 18g
- Carbohydrates: 50g
- Fat: 16g
- Fiber: 6g
- Sugar: 2g

Number of Servings:

- **4 servings**

Cooking Time:

- **20 minutes**

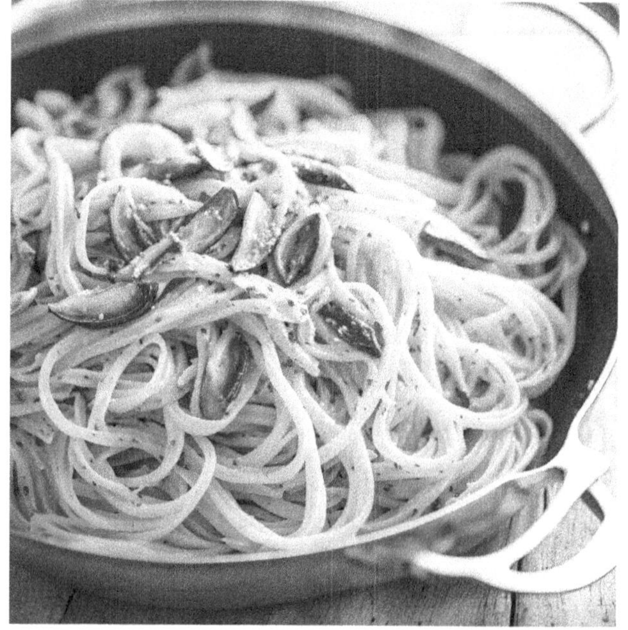

25. Baked Lemon Sole with Capers

Ingredients:

- 4 sole fillets (6 ounces each)
- 2 tablespoons olive oil
- 1 lemon, thinly sliced
- 2 tablespoons capers, rinsed
- 1/4 teaspoon black pepper
- Fresh parsley for garnish (optional)

Instructions:

1. Preheat the oven to 375°F (190°C).
2. Place the sole fillets in a baking dish and drizzle with olive oil.
3. Arrange the lemon slices and capers over the sole fillets. Sprinkle with black pepper.
4. Bake for 15-20 minutes, until the fish is opaque and flakes easily with a fork.
5. Garnish with fresh parsley if desired.
6. Serve immediately.

Nutrition Info per Serving:

- Calories: 220
- Protein: 28g
- Carbohydrates: 4g
- Fat: 10g
- Fiber: 1g
- Sugar: 1g

Number of Servings:

- **4 servings**

Cooking Time:

- **20 minutes**

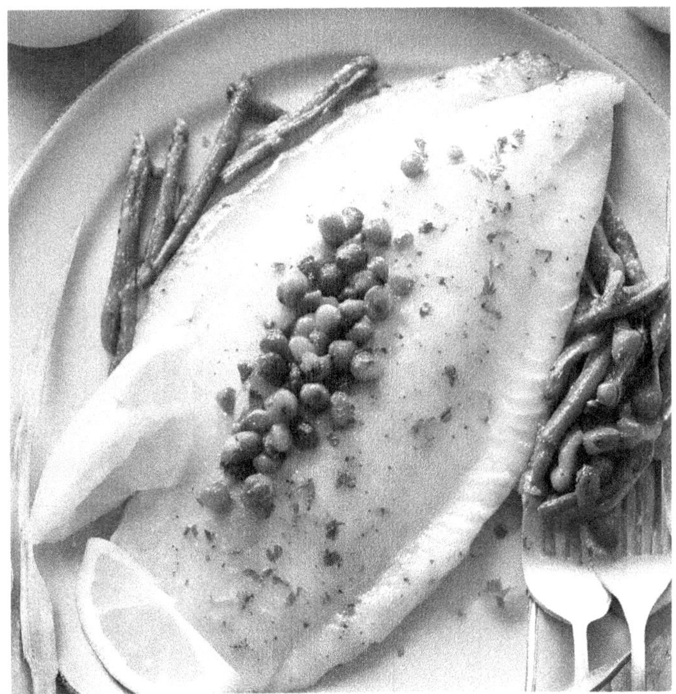

26. Snapper Veracruz

Ingredients:

- 4 snapper fillets (6 ounces each)
- 2 tablespoons olive oil
- 1 large onion, diced
- 2 cloves garlic, minced
- 1 can (14.5 ounces) diced tomatoes
- 1/2 cup green olives, sliced
- 1/4 cup capers, rinsed
- 1/2 teaspoon dried oregano
- 1/4 teaspoon black pepper
- 1 tablespoon fresh lime juice
- Fresh cilantro for garnish (optional)

Instructions:

1. Preheat the oven to 375°F (190°C).
2. Heat 1 tablespoon of olive oil in a large skillet over medium heat. Add the onion and garlic, and cook until softened, about 5 minutes.
3. Stir in the diced tomatoes, green olives, capers, oregano, and black pepper. Cook for another 5 minutes until the sauce is heated through.
4. Place the snapper fillets in a baking dish and pour the tomato mixture over the top.
5. Drizzle with the remaining 1 tablespoon of olive oil and bake for 20-25 minutes, until the fish is opaque and flakes easily with a fork.
6. Garnish with fresh cilantro and a squeeze of lime juice if desired.
7. Serve immediately.

Nutrition Info per Serving:

- Calories: 300
- Protein: 32g
- Carbohydrates: 8g
- Fat: 16g
- Fiber: 3g
- Sugar: 4g

Number of Servings:

- **4 servings**

Cooking Time:

- **30 minutes**

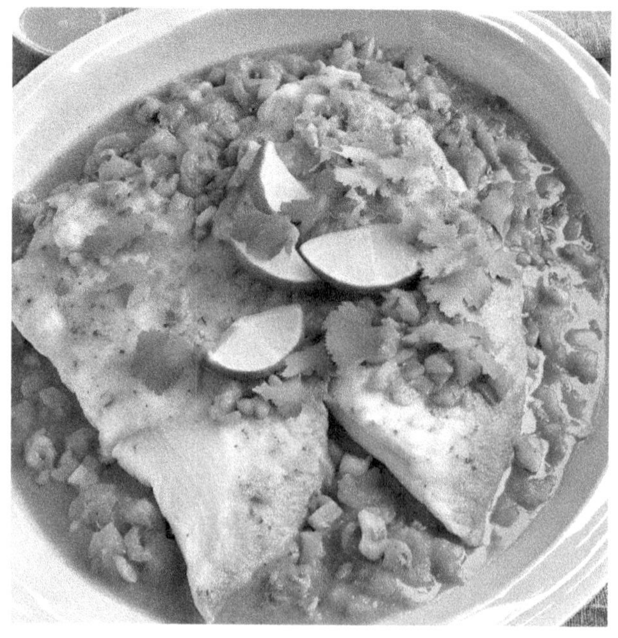

27. Grilled Swordfish with Herb Salad

Ingredients:

- 4 swordfish steaks (6 ounces each)
- 2 tablespoons olive oil
- 1/4 teaspoon black pepper
- 1/4 cup fresh parsley, chopped
- 1/4 cup fresh mint, chopped
- 1/4 cup fresh basil, chopped
- 1/4 cup fresh cilantro, chopped
- 1 tablespoon lemon juice
- 1 teaspoon honey

Instructions:

1. Preheat the grill to medium-high heat.
2. Brush the swordfish steaks with 1 tablespoon of olive oil and sprinkle with black pepper.
3. Grill the swordfish for 4-5 minutes per side, until the fish is opaque and flakes easily with a fork.
4. In a small bowl, combine the parsley, mint, basil, cilantro, lemon juice, honey, and the remaining 1 tablespoon of olive oil to make the herb salad.
5. Serve the grilled swordfish topped with the herb salad.
6. Serve immediately.

Nutrition Info per Serving:

- Calories: 350
- Protein: 34g
- Carbohydrates: 6g
- Fat: 20g
- Fiber: 2g
- Sugar: 3g

Number of Servings:

- **4 servings**

Cooking Time:

- **15 minutes**

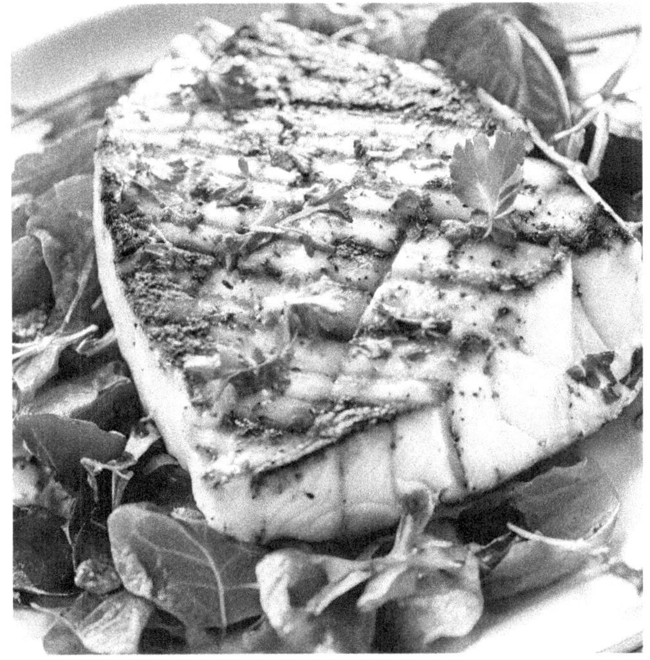

28. Garlic Butter Shrimp Pasta

Ingredients:

- 1 pound large shrimp, peeled and deveined
- 8 ounces whole wheat spaghetti
- 2 tablespoons olive oil
- 2 tablespoons unsalted butter
- 4 cloves garlic, minced
- 1/4 teaspoon red pepper flakes
- 1/4 cup grated Parmesan cheese (optional)
- 1/4 cup chopped fresh parsley
- 1 tablespoon lemon juice

Instructions:

1. Cook the spaghetti according to package instructions. Drain and set aside.
2. In a large skillet, heat the olive oil and butter over medium heat. Add the garlic and red pepper flakes, and cook for 1 minute until fragrant.
3. Add the shrimp to the skillet and cook for 3-4 minutes, until pink and opaque.
4. Add the cooked spaghetti to the skillet and toss to coat in the garlic butter sauce.
5. Stir in the Parmesan cheese (if using), fresh parsley, and lemon juice.
6. Serve immediately.

Nutrition Info per Serving:

- Calories: 400
- Protein: 30g
- Carbohydrates: 45g
- Fat: 15g
- Fiber: 6g
- Sugar: 2g

Number of Servings:

- **4 servings**

Cooking Time:

- **20 minutes**

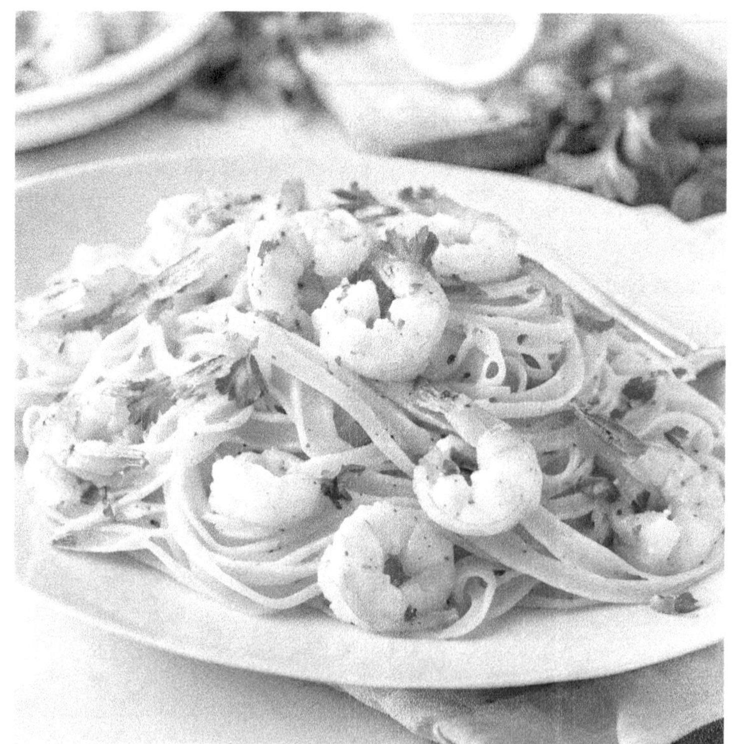

29. Fried Calamari with Marinara Sauce

Ingredients:

- 1 pound calamari rings
- 1 cup whole wheat flour
- 1/4 teaspoon black pepper
- 2 eggs, beaten
- 1 cup whole wheat breadcrumbs
- 2 cups olive oil (for frying)
- 1 cup marinara sauce (for serving)
- Lemon wedges (optional, for serving)

Instructions:

1. Heat the olive oil in a large pot or deep fryer to 350°F (175°C).
2. In a shallow dish, mix the flour and black pepper.
3. In another shallow dish, place the beaten eggs.
4. In a third shallow dish, place the breadcrumbs.
5. Dredge the calamari rings in the flour, then dip in the beaten eggs, and coat with breadcrumbs.
6. Fry the calamari in batches for 2-3 minutes until golden brown and crispy. Drain on paper towels.
7. Serve with marinara sauce and lemon wedges if desired.

Nutrition Info per Serving:

- Calories: 400
- Protein: 20g
- Carbohydrates: 30g
- Fat: 20g
- Fiber: 4g
- Sugar: 3g

Number of Servings:

- **4 servings**

Cooking Time:

- **15 minutes**

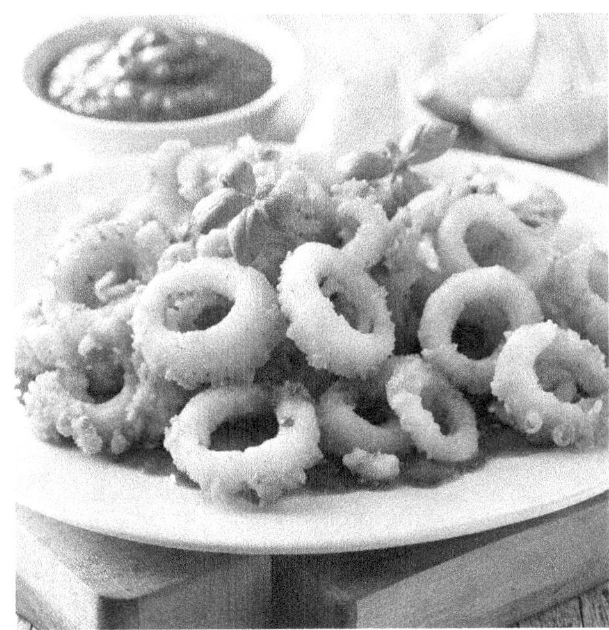

30. Perch with Creamy Dill Sauce

Ingredients:

- 4 perch fillets (6 ounces each)
- 2 tablespoons olive oil
- 1/4 teaspoon black pepper
- 1/2 cup plain Greek yogurt
- 1 tablespoon fresh dill, chopped
- 1 tablespoon lemon juice
- 1 garlic clove, minced

Instructions:

1. Heat olive oil in a large skillet over medium heat.
2. Sprinkle the perch fillets with black pepper and cook for 3-4 minutes per side until opaque and cooked through.
3. In a small bowl, mix the Greek yogurt, dill, lemon juice, and minced garlic to make the creamy dill sauce.
4. Serve the perch fillets with the creamy dill sauce on top.

Nutrition Info per Serving:

- Calories: 250
- Protein: 30g
- Carbohydrates: 5g
- Fat: 12g
- Fiber: 0g
- Sugar: 2g

Number of Servings:

- **4 servings**

Cooking Time:

- **10 minutes**

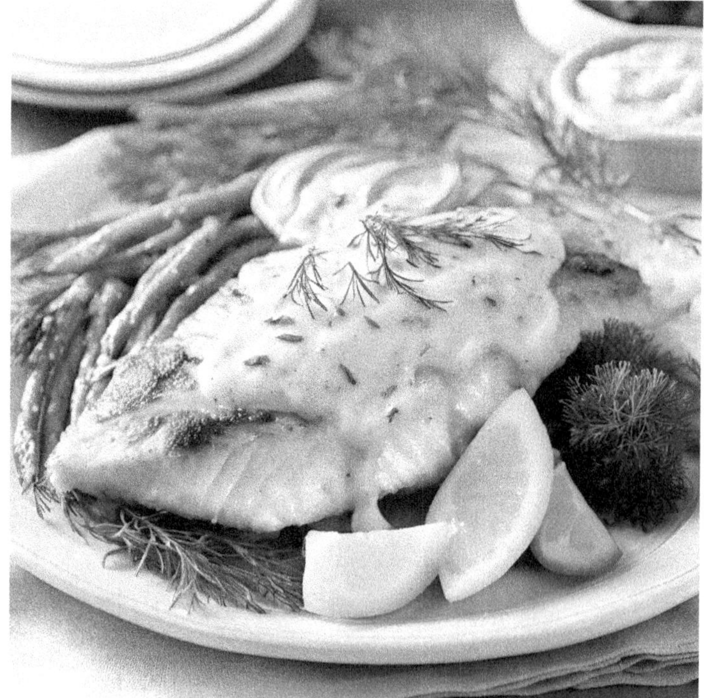

31. Steamer Clams with Lemon

Ingredients:

- 2 pounds steamer clams, scrubbed
- 2 tablespoons olive oil
- 4 cloves garlic, minced
- 1 cup low-sodium vegetable broth
- 1/4 cup white wine (optional)
- 1 lemon, juiced
- 1/4 teaspoon black pepper
- Fresh parsley for garnish (optional)

Instructions:

1. Heat olive oil in a large pot over medium heat. Add the garlic and cook for 1 minute until fragrant.
2. Add the vegetable broth, white wine (if using), lemon juice, and black pepper. Bring to a boil.
3. Add the clams, cover, and cook for 5-7 minutes until the clams open.
4. Discard any clams that do not open.
5. Garnish with fresh parsley if desired and serve immediately.

Nutrition Info per Serving:

- Calories: 200
- Protein: 24g
- Carbohydrates: 8g
- Fat: 8g
- Fiber: 1g
- Sugar: 0g

Number of Servings:

- 4 servings

Cooking Time:

- 15 minutes

32. Pan-Fried Mackerel with Lemon

Ingredients:

- 4 mackerel fillets (6 ounces each)
- 2 tablespoons olive oil
- 1/4 teaspoon black pepper
- 1 lemon, thinly sliced
- 1 tablespoon fresh parsley, chopped (optional)

Instructions:

1. Heat olive oil in a large skillet over medium-high heat.
2. Sprinkle the mackerel fillets with black pepper and place them skin-side down in the skillet.
3. Cook for 3-4 minutes until the skin is crispy, then flip and cook for another 2-3 minutes until cooked through.
4. Serve with lemon slices and garnish with fresh parsley if desired.

Nutrition Info per Serving:

- Calories: 350
- Protein: 30g
- Carbohydrates: 3g
- Fat: 24g
- Fiber: 1g
- Sugar: 0g

Number of Servings:

- **4 servings**

Cooking Time:

- **10 minutes**

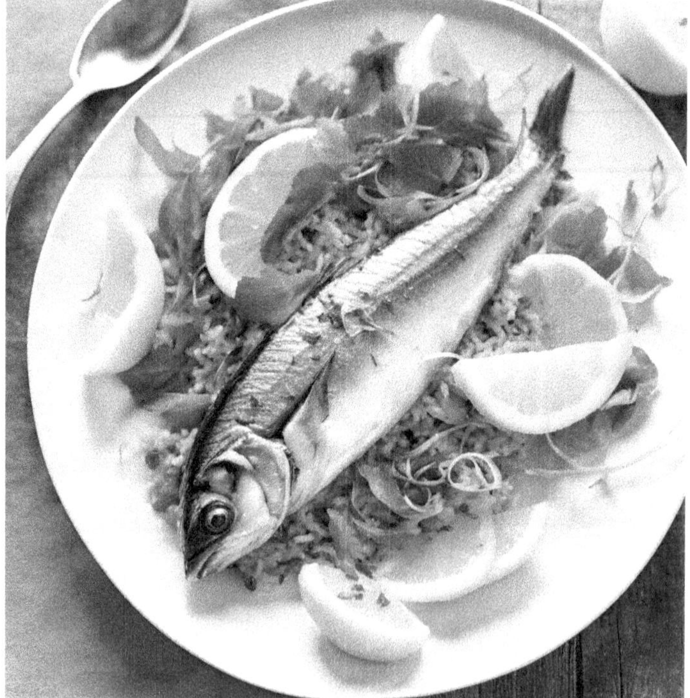

33. Pasta with Smoked Mackerel

Ingredients:

- 8 ounces whole wheat pasta
- 2 tablespoons olive oil
- 1 onion, finely diced
- 2 cloves garlic, minced
- 1/2 cup sun-dried tomatoes, chopped
- 1/2 cup low-sodium vegetable broth
- 1 cup smoked mackerel, flaked
- 1 tablespoon lemon juice
- 1/4 teaspoon black pepper
- 1/4 cup fresh parsley, chopped

Instructions:

1. Cook the pasta according to package instructions. Drain and set aside.
2. In a large skillet, heat olive oil over medium heat. Add the onion and garlic, and cook until softened, about 5 minutes.
3. Add the sun-dried tomatoes and vegetable broth, and cook for another 3 minutes.
4. Stir in the smoked mackerel, lemon juice, and black pepper. Cook until heated through.
5. Add the cooked pasta to the skillet and toss to combine.
6. Serve topped with fresh parsley.

Nutrition Info per Serving:

- Calories: 400
- Protein: 25g
- Carbohydrates: 50g
- Fat: 12g
- Fiber: 6g
- Sugar: 5g

Number of Servings:

- **4 servings**

Cooking Time:

- **20 minutes**

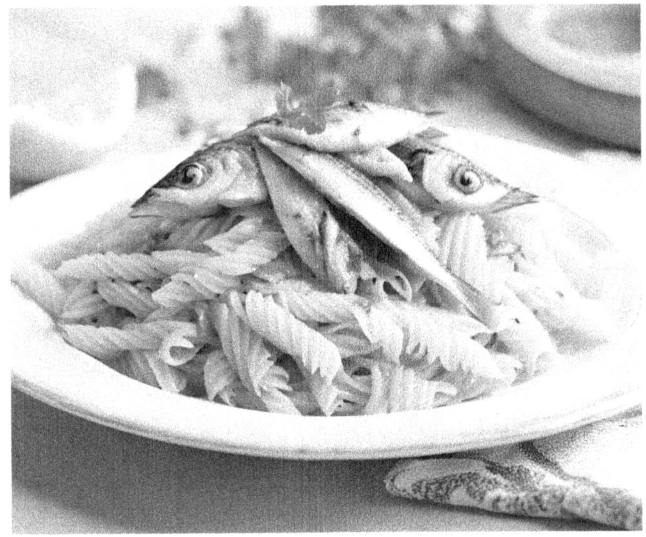

Poultry Recipes

1. One-Pot Chicken and Vegetables

Ingredients:

- 4 bone-in chicken thighs
- 2 tablespoons olive oil
- 1 large onion, diced
- 3 cloves garlic, minced
- 2 carrots, sliced
- 2 celery stalks, sliced
- 1 red bell pepper, chopped
- 1 cup baby potatoes, halved
- 1 teaspoon dried thyme
- 1/2 teaspoon dried rosemary
- 1/4 teaspoon black pepper
- 2 cups low-sodium chicken broth
- 1 cup green beans, trimmed

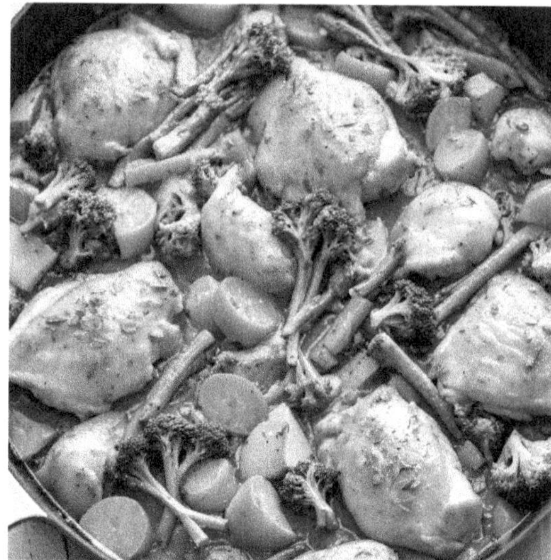

Instructions:

1. Heat olive oil in a large pot over medium heat. Add the chicken thighs and brown on both sides, about 5-7 minutes per side. Remove from the pot and set aside.
2. In the same pot, add the onion and garlic, and cook until softened, about 3-4 minutes.
3. Add the carrots, celery, bell pepper, and baby potatoes. Cook for another 5 minutes.
4. Stir in the thyme, rosemary, and black pepper.
5. Return the chicken thighs to the pot and pour in the chicken broth.
6. Bring to a boil, then reduce heat and simmer for 30 minutes, until the chicken is cooked through and the vegetables are tender.
7. Add the green beans and cook for an additional 5 minutes.
8. Serve immediately.

Nutrition Info per Serving:

- Calories: 350
- Protein: 25g
- Carbohydrates: 20g
- Fat: 18g
- Fiber: 5g
- Sugar: 6g

Number of Servings:

- **4 servings**

Cooking Time:

- **50 minutes**

2. Chicken Provençal

Ingredients:

- 4 boneless, skinless chicken breasts
- 2 tablespoons olive oil
- 1 large onion, diced
- 3 cloves garlic, minced
- 1 can (14.5 ounces) diced tomatoes
- 1/2 cup pitted Kalamata olives
- 1/2 cup low-sodium chicken broth
- 1 teaspoon dried thyme
- 1 teaspoon dried oregano
- 1/4 teaspoon black pepper
- Fresh basil for garnish (optional)

Instructions:

1. Heat olive oil in a large skillet over medium heat. Add the chicken breasts and brown on both sides, about 5-7 minutes per side. Remove from the skillet and set aside.
2. In the same skillet, add the onion and garlic, and cook until softened, about 3-4 minutes.
3. Stir in the diced tomatoes, Kalamata olives, chicken broth, thyme, oregano, and black pepper.
4. Return the chicken breasts to the skillet, spooning some of the sauce over the top.
5. Cover and simmer for 20-25 minutes, until the chicken is cooked through.
6. Garnish with fresh basil if desired.
7. Serve immediately.

Nutrition Info per Serving:

- Calories: 300
- Protein: 32g
- Carbohydrates: 12g
- Fat: 15g
- Fiber: 3g
- Sugar: 6g

Number of Servings:

- **4 servings**

Cooking Time:

- **35 minutes**

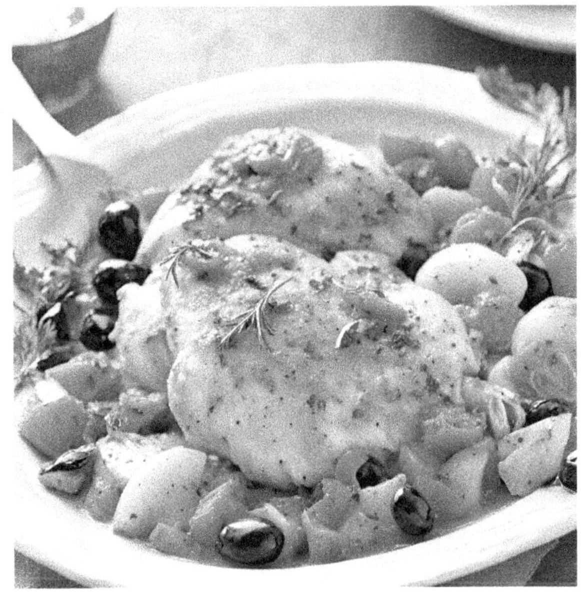

3. Lemon Thyme Turkey Cutlets

Ingredients:

- 4 turkey cutlets (about 4 ounces each)
- 2 tablespoons olive oil
- 1/4 teaspoon black pepper
- 2 cloves garlic, minced
- 1 tablespoon fresh thyme leaves
- 1 lemon, zested and juiced
- 1/2 cup low-sodium chicken broth
- Fresh parsley for garnish (optional)

Instructions:

1. Heat olive oil in a large skillet over medium heat.
2. Sprinkle the turkey cutlets with black pepper and add to the skillet. Cook for 3-4 minutes per side, until golden brown and cooked through. Remove from the skillet and set aside.
3. In the same skillet, add the garlic and thyme, and cook for 1 minute until fragrant.
4. Stir in the lemon zest, lemon juice, and chicken broth. Bring to a simmer.
5. Return the turkey cutlets to the skillet and spoon the sauce over them. Cook for an additional 2-3 minutes.
6. Garnish with fresh parsley if desired.
7. Serve immediately.

Nutrition Info per Serving:

- Calories: 220
- Protein: 28g
- Carbohydrates: 4g
- Fat: 10g
- Fiber: 1g
- Sugar: 1g

Number of Servings:

- **4 servings**

Cooking Time:

- **15 minutes**

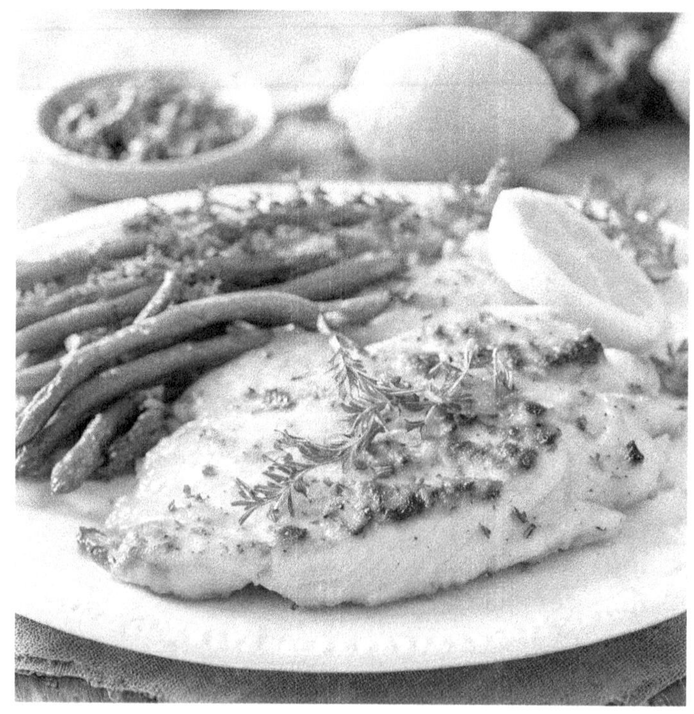

4. Chicken Paillard

Ingredients:

- 4 boneless, skinless chicken breasts
- 2 tablespoons olive oil
- 1/4 teaspoon black pepper
- 2 cloves garlic, minced
- 1 lemon, zested and juiced
- 1 tablespoon fresh parsley, chopped
- 1 tablespoon fresh basil, chopped
- 1 cup arugula
- Lemon wedges (optional, for serving)

Instructions:

1. Pound the chicken breasts to an even thickness using a meat mallet or rolling pin.
2. Heat olive oil in a large skillet over medium-high heat.
3. Sprinkle the chicken breasts with black pepper and add to the skillet. Cook for 3-4 minutes per side until golden brown and cooked through. Remove from the skillet and set aside.
4. In the same skillet, add the garlic and cook for 1 minute until fragrant.
5. Stir in the lemon zest and lemon juice. Cook for an additional 1 minute.
6. Pour the sauce over the chicken breasts and garnish with fresh parsley and basil.
7. Serve the chicken paillard on a bed of arugula with lemon wedges on the side.
8. Serve immediately.

Nutrition Info per Serving:

- Calories: 250
- Protein: 30g
- Carbohydrates: 4g
- Fat: 12g
- Fiber: 1g
- Sugar: 1g

Number of Servings:

- **4 servings**

Cooking Time:

- **15 minutes**

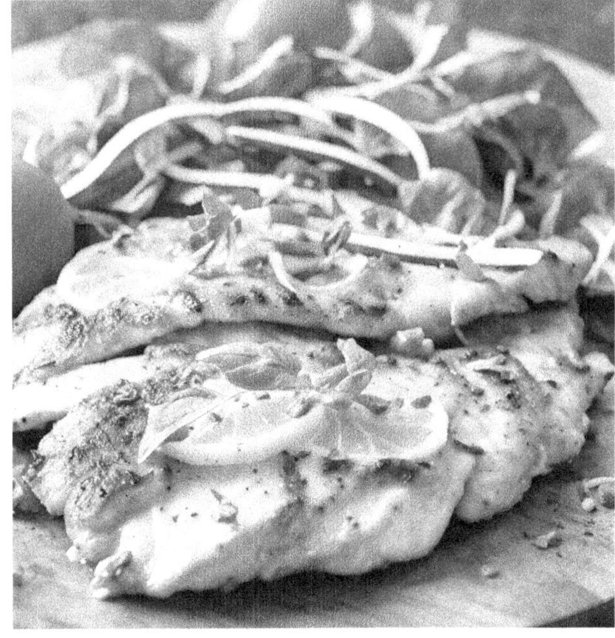

5. Pan-Seared Duck Breast

Ingredients:

- 4 duck breasts (6 ounces each)
- 2 tablespoons olive oil
- 1/4 teaspoon black pepper
- 1/4 teaspoon dried thyme
- 2 cloves garlic, minced
- 1 tablespoon balsamic vinegar
- 1 tablespoon honey
- 1/4 cup low-sodium chicken broth

Instructions:

1. Score the skin of the duck breasts in a crosshatch pattern.
2. Sprinkle the duck breasts with black pepper and dried thyme.
3. Heat a large skillet over medium-high heat. Add the duck breasts skin-side down and cook for 5-7 minutes until the skin is crispy and golden brown. Flip and cook for another 3-4 minutes for medium-rare.
4. Remove the duck breasts from the skillet and set aside to rest.
5. In the same skillet, add the garlic and cook for 1 minute until fragrant.
6. Stir in the balsamic vinegar, honey, and chicken broth. Cook for 2-3 minutes until the sauce has reduced and thickened slightly.
7. Slice the duck breasts and serve with the balsamic reduction sauce.

Nutrition Info per Serving:

- Calories: 350
- Protein: 28g
- Carbohydrates: 5g
- Fat: 22g
- Fiber: 0g
- Sugar: 3g

Number of Servings:

- **4 servings**

Cooking Time:

- **20 minutes**

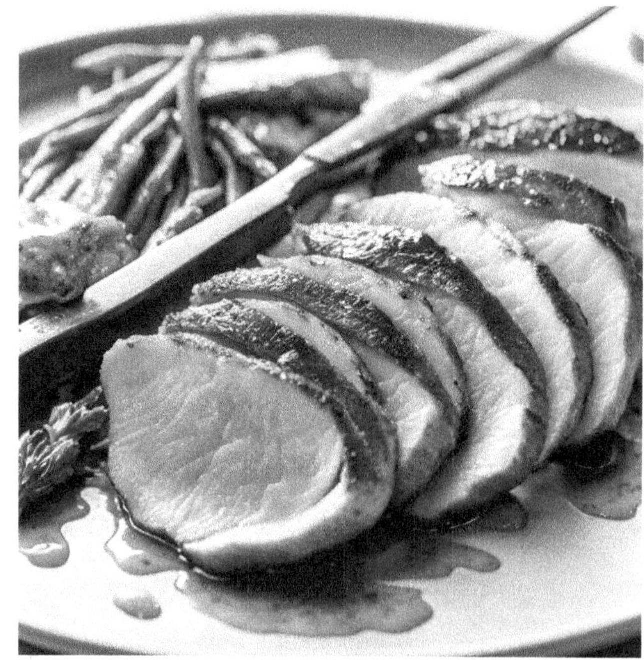

6. Mediterranean Turkey Patties

Ingredients:

- 1 pound ground turkey
- 1/4 cup finely chopped red onion
- 1/4 cup chopped fresh parsley
- 1/4 cup chopped kalamata olives
- 1/4 cup crumbled feta cheese
- 1 teaspoon dried oregano
- 1/4 teaspoon black pepper
- 1 tablespoon olive oil
- 1 tablespoon lemon juice

Instructions:

1. In a large bowl, combine the ground turkey, red onion, parsley, kalamata olives, feta cheese, oregano, black pepper, and lemon juice. Mix until well combined.
2. Form the mixture into 4 patties.
3. Heat the olive oil in a large skillet over medium heat. Add the patties and cook for 5-7 minutes per side, until fully cooked through.
4. Serve immediately.

Nutrition Info per Serving:

- Calories: 250
- Protein: 28g
- Carbohydrates: 3g
- Fat: 14g
- Fiber: 1g
- Sugar: 1g

Number of Servings:

- **4 servings**

Cooking Time:

- **15 minutes**

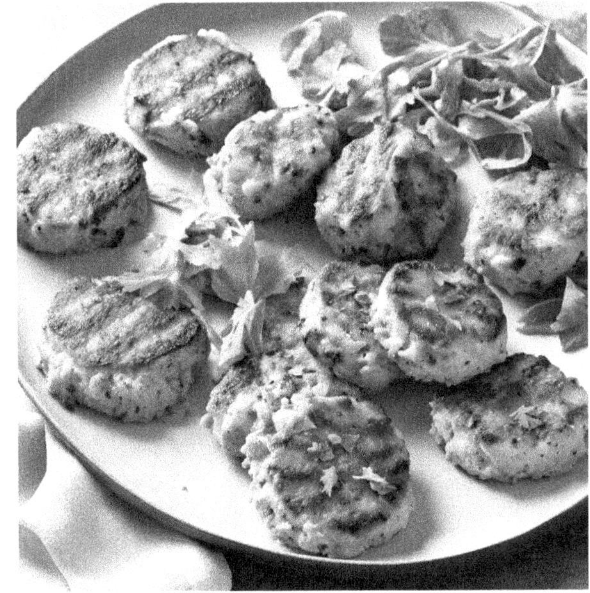

7. Sesame Ginger Chicken

Ingredients:

- 4 boneless, skinless chicken breasts
- 2 tablespoons olive oil
- 1 tablespoon grated fresh ginger
- 2 cloves garlic, minced
- 1/4 cup low-sodium soy sauce
- 1 tablespoon honey
- 1 tablespoon rice vinegar
- 1 tablespoon sesame seeds
- 1 green onion, sliced (optional for garnish)

Instructions:

1. Heat the olive oil in a large skillet over medium heat.
2. Add the chicken breasts and cook for 5-7 minutes per side until golden brown and cooked through. Remove from the skillet and set aside.
3. In the same skillet, add the ginger and garlic. Cook for 1 minute until fragrant.
4. Stir in the soy sauce, honey, and rice vinegar. Cook for 2-3 minutes until the sauce thickens slightly.
5. Return the chicken to the skillet and coat with the sauce. Cook for an additional 2 minutes.
6. Sprinkle with sesame seeds and garnish with green onion if desired.
7. Serve immediately.

Nutrition Info per Serving:

- Calories: 280
- Protein: 30g
- Carbohydrates: 10g
- Fat: 12g
- Fiber: 1g
- Sugar: 5g

Number of Servings:

- **4 servings**

Cooking Time:

- **20 minutes**

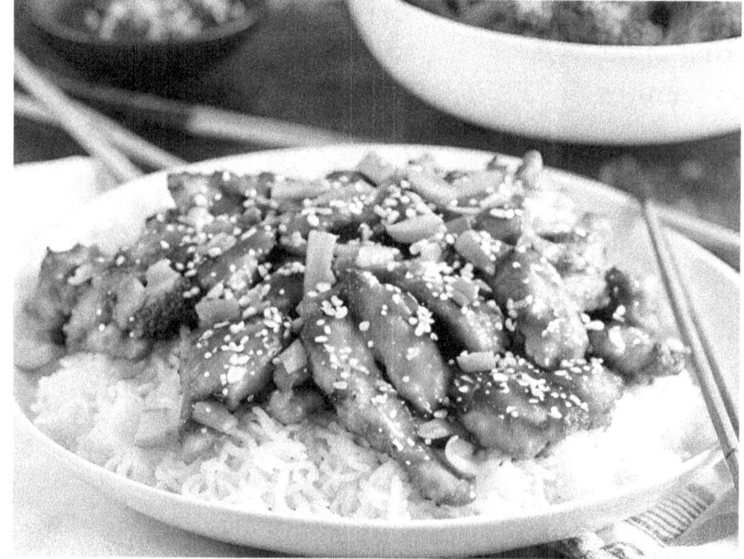

8. Chicken Minestrone Soup

Ingredients:

- 2 boneless, skinless chicken breasts, diced
- 2 tablespoons olive oil
- 1 large onion, diced
- 3 cloves garlic, minced
- 2 carrots, sliced
- 2 celery stalks, sliced
- 1 zucchini, diced
- 1 can (14.5 ounces) diced tomatoes
- 4 cups low-sodium chicken broth
- 1 can (15 ounces) cannellini beans, rinsed and drained
- 1 teaspoon dried basil
- 1 teaspoon dried oregano
- 1/4 teaspoon black pepper
- 1 cup whole wheat pasta

Instructions:

1. Heat the olive oil in a large pot over medium heat. Add the chicken and cook until browned, about 5 minutes.
2. Add the onion and garlic, and cook until softened, about 3-4 minutes.
3. Stir in the carrots, celery, and zucchini. Cook for another 5 minutes.
4. Add the diced tomatoes, chicken broth, cannellini beans, basil, oregano, and black pepper. Bring to a boil.
5. Reduce heat and simmer for 20 minutes.
6. Add the pasta and cook for an additional 10 minutes until tender.
7. Serve immediately.

Nutrition Info per Serving:

- Calories: 300
- Protein: 25g
- Carbohydrates: 35g
- Fat: 8g
- Fiber: 6g
- Sugar: 8g

Number of Servings:

- **4 servings**

Cooking Time:

- **35 minutes**

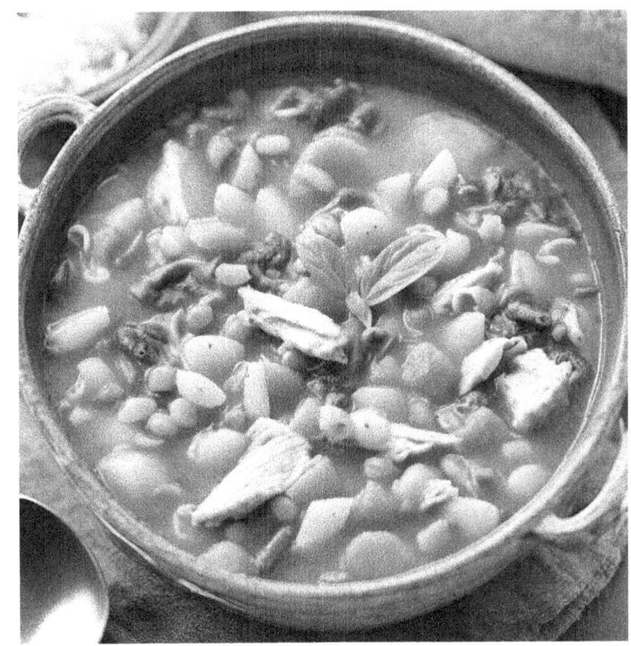

9. Turkey and Quinoa Stuffed Zucchini

Ingredients:

- 4 large zucchini, halved lengthwise and seeds scooped out
- 1/2 pound ground turkey
- 1/2 cup cooked quinoa
- 1 small onion, diced
- 2 cloves garlic, minced
- 1/2 cup diced tomatoes
- 1/4 cup grated Parmesan cheese (optional)
- 1 teaspoon dried oregano
- 1/4 teaspoon black pepper
- 1 tablespoon olive oil
- Fresh parsley for garnish (optional)

Instructions:

1. Preheat the oven to 375°F (190°C).
2. Heat the olive oil in a skillet over medium heat. Add the onion and garlic, and cook until softened, about 3-4 minutes.
3. Add the ground turkey and cook until browned, about 5-7 minutes.
4. Stir in the cooked quinoa, diced tomatoes, oregano, and black pepper.
5. Stuff the zucchini halves with the turkey mixture and place in a baking dish.
6. Sprinkle with Parmesan cheese if using.
7. Bake for 20-25 minutes until the zucchini is tender.
8. Garnish with fresh parsley if desired.
9. Serve immediately.

Nutrition Info per Serving:

- Calories: 220
- Protein: 20g
- Carbohydrates: 15g
- Fat: 10g
- Fiber: 4g
- Sugar: 5g

Number of Servings:

- 4 servings

Cooking Time:

- 30 minutes

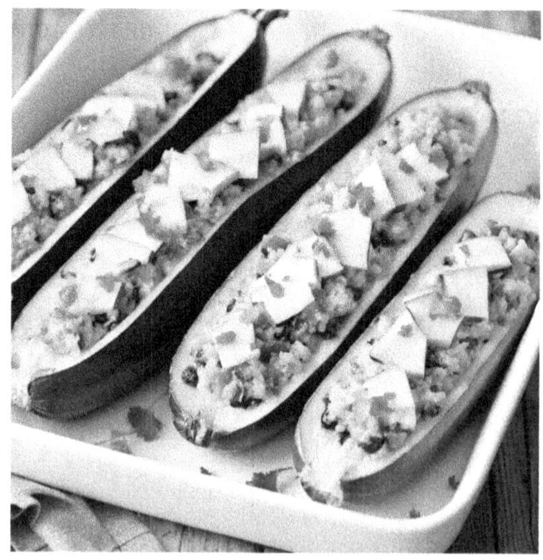

10. Chicken Tenders with Almond Crust

Ingredients:

- 1 pound chicken tenders
- 1/2 cup almond flour
- 1/2 cup whole wheat breadcrumbs
- 1/4 teaspoon black pepper
- 1 teaspoon garlic powder
- 1 teaspoon paprika
- 2 eggs, beaten
- 2 tablespoons olive oil

Instructions:

1. Preheat the oven to 375°F (190°C) and line a baking sheet with parchment paper.
2. In a shallow dish, combine almond flour, breadcrumbs, black pepper, garlic powder, and paprika.
3. Dip each chicken tender into the beaten eggs, then coat with the almond flour mixture.
4. Heat the olive oil in a large skillet over medium heat. Cook the chicken tenders for 2-3 minutes per side until golden brown.
5. Transfer the chicken tenders to the prepared baking sheet and bake for 15-20 minutes until cooked through.
6. Serve immediately.

Nutrition Info per Serving:

- Calories: 320
- Protein: 30g
- Carbohydrates: 10g
- Fat: 18g
- Fiber: 3g
- Sugar: 1g

Number of Servings:

- **4 servings**

Cooking Time:

- **30 minutes**

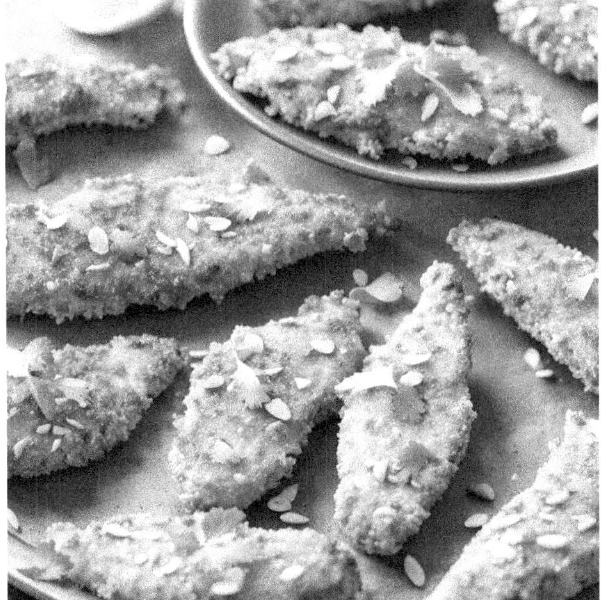

11. Garlic and Herb Roasted Turkey

Ingredients:

- 1 whole turkey (12-14 pounds)
- 1/2 cup olive oil
- 6 cloves garlic, minced
- 2 tablespoons fresh rosemary, chopped
- 2 tablespoons fresh thyme, chopped
- 1 tablespoon fresh sage, chopped
- 1/4 teaspoon black pepper
- 1 lemon, halved

Instructions:

1. Preheat the oven to 325°F (165°C).
2. In a small bowl, mix the olive oil, garlic, rosemary, thyme, sage, and black pepper.
3. Rub the herb mixture all over the turkey, including under the skin.
4. Place the lemon halves inside the turkey cavity.
5. Roast the turkey on a rack in a roasting pan for 3-3.5 hours, or until the internal temperature reaches 165°F (74°C).
6. Let the turkey rest for 20 minutes before carving.
7. Serve immediately.

Nutrition Info per Serving:

- Calories: 450
- Protein: 65g
- Carbohydrates: 2g
- Fat: 20g
- Fiber: 1g
- Sugar: 0g

Number of Servings:

- **12 servings**

Cooking Time:

- **3.5 hours**

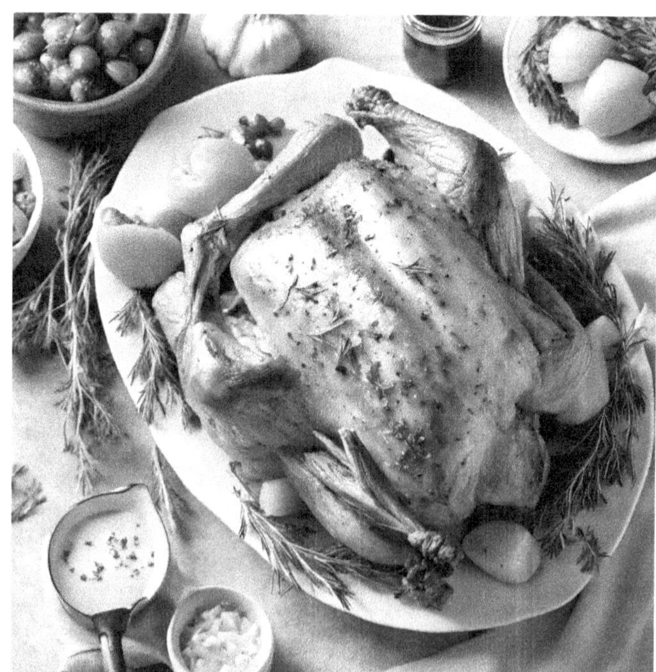

12. Chicken and Pea Risotto

Ingredients:

- 1 pound boneless, skinless chicken breasts, diced
- 1 cup Arborio rice
- 4 cups low-sodium chicken broth
- 1 cup frozen peas
- 1/2 cup grated Parmesan cheese (optional)
- 1 small onion, finely diced
- 2 cloves garlic, minced
- 2 tablespoons olive oil
- 1/4 teaspoon black pepper
- 1/4 cup white wine (optional)
- 1 tablespoon fresh parsley, chopped (optional)

Instructions:

1. Heat the chicken broth in a saucepan and keep it warm over low heat.
2. In a large skillet, heat 1 tablespoon of olive oil over medium heat. Add the diced chicken and cook until browned and cooked through, about 5-7 minutes. Remove from the skillet and set aside.
3. In the same skillet, heat the remaining 1 tablespoon of olive oil. Add the onion and garlic, and cook until softened, about 3-4 minutes.
4. Add the Arborio rice and cook, stirring frequently, for 2 minutes.
5. Pour in the white wine (if using) and cook until it is mostly absorbed.
6. Begin adding the warm broth, one ladle at a time, stirring constantly and waiting until the liquid is absorbed before adding more. Continue until the rice is creamy and cooked through, about 20 minutes.
7. Stir in the cooked chicken, peas, Parmesan cheese (if using), and black pepper. Cook for an additional 5 minutes until heated through.
8. Garnish with fresh parsley if desired.
9. Serve immediately.

Nutrition Info per Serving:

- Calories: 350
- Protein: 30g
- Carbohydrates: 40g
- Fat: 10g
- Fiber: 3g
- Sugar: 3g

Number of Servings:

- **4 servings**

Cooking Time:

- **30 minutes**

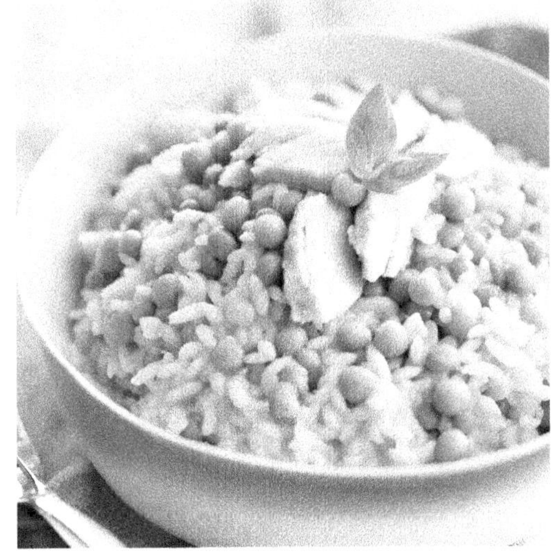

13. Chicken Fajitas

Ingredients:

- 1 pound boneless, skinless chicken breasts, thinly sliced
- 1 red bell pepper, sliced
- 1 green bell pepper, sliced
- 1 yellow bell pepper, sliced
- 1 large onion, sliced
- 2 tablespoons olive oil
- 1 teaspoon ground cumin
- 1 teaspoon paprika
- 1/2 teaspoon garlic powder
- 1/4 teaspoon black pepper
- 8 small whole wheat tortillas
- Fresh cilantro and lime wedges for serving (optional)

Instructions:

1. Heat the olive oil in a large skillet over medium heat.
2. Add the chicken slices, cumin, paprika, garlic powder, and black pepper. Cook until the chicken is browned and cooked through, about 5-7 minutes.
3. Add the bell peppers and onion to the skillet. Cook until the vegetables are tender, about 5-7 minutes.
4. Warm the tortillas in a separate skillet or microwave.
5. Serve the chicken and vegetable mixture in the tortillas. Garnish with fresh cilantro and lime wedges if desired.
6. Serve immediately.

Nutrition Info per Serving:

- Calories: 350
- Protein: 28g
- Carbohydrates: 30g
- Fat: 12g
- Fiber: 6g
- Sugar: 5g

Number of Servings:

- **4 servings**

Cooking Time:

- **20 minutes**

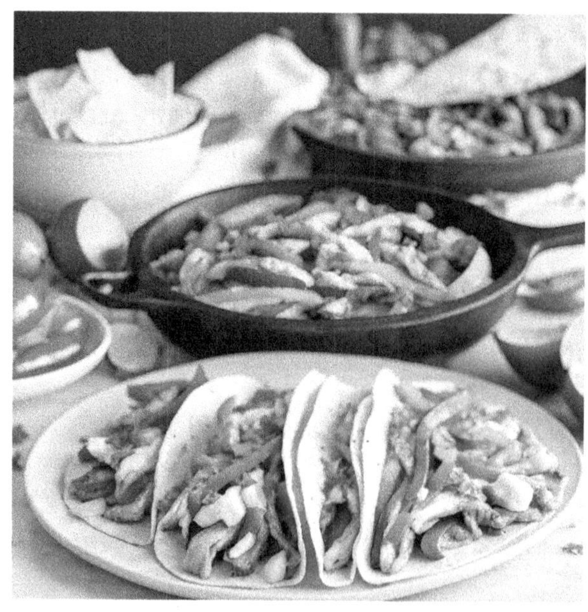

14. Turkey Sloppy Joes

Ingredients:

- 1 pound ground turkey
- 1 small onion, diced
- 1 green bell pepper, diced
- 2 cloves garlic, minced
- 1 can (8 ounces) tomato sauce
- 1/4 cup tomato paste
- 1 tablespoon Worcestershire sauce
- 1 tablespoon honey
- 1/4 teaspoon black pepper
- 4 whole wheat hamburger buns

Instructions:

1. Heat a large skillet over medium heat. Add the ground turkey, onion, bell pepper, and garlic. Cook until the turkey is browned and the vegetables are softened, about 7-10 minutes.
2. Stir in the tomato sauce, tomato paste, Worcestershire sauce, honey, and black pepper. Cook for an additional 5-7 minutes, until the mixture is thickened.
3. Serve the turkey mixture on whole wheat hamburger buns.
4. Serve immediately.

Nutrition Info per Serving:

- Calories: 300
- Protein: 28g
- Carbohydrates: 30g
- Fat: 8g
- Fiber: 4g
- Sugar: 8g

Number of Servings:

- **4 servings**

Cooking Time:

- **20 minutes**

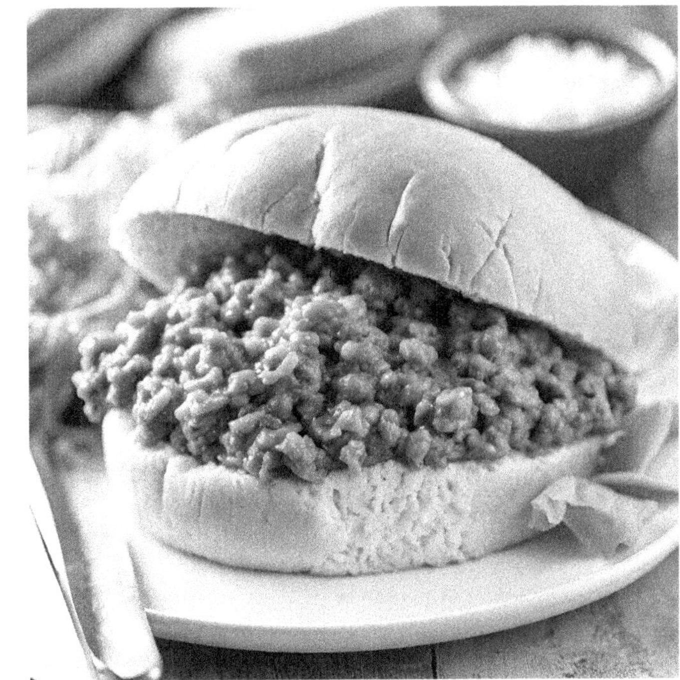

15. Smoked Paprika Chicken

Ingredients:

- 4 boneless, skinless chicken breasts
- 2 tablespoons olive oil
- 2 teaspoons smoked paprika
- 1 teaspoon garlic powder
- 1/4 teaspoon black pepper
- 1 lemon, sliced
- Fresh parsley for garnish (optional)

Instructions:

1. Preheat the oven to 375°F (190°C).
2. In a small bowl, mix olive oil, smoked paprika, garlic powder, and black pepper.
3. Rub the spice mixture all over the chicken breasts.
4. Place the chicken breasts in a baking dish and top with lemon slices.
5. Bake for 25-30 minutes, until the chicken is cooked through and juices run clear.
6. Garnish with fresh parsley if desired.
7. Serve immediately.

Nutrition Info per Serving:

- Calories: 280
- Protein: 30g
- Carbohydrates: 2g
- Fat: 16g
- Fiber: 1g
- Sugar: 1g

Number of Servings:

- 4 servings

Cooking Time:

- 30 minutes

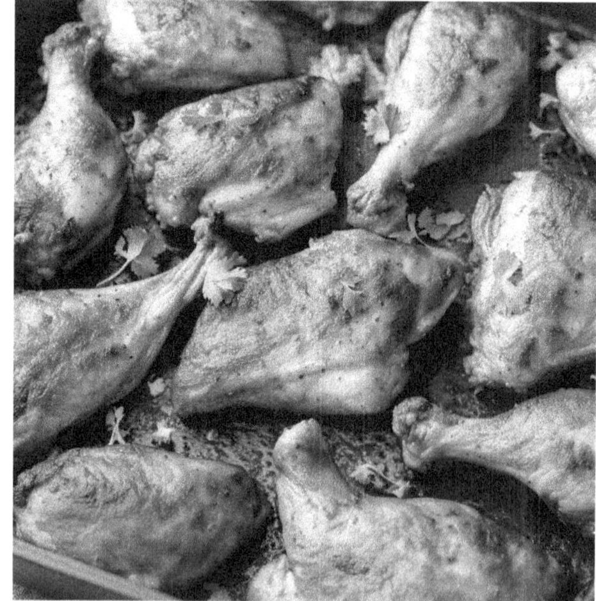

16. Roast Chicken with Root Vegetables

Ingredients:

- 1 whole chicken (4-5 pounds)
- 4 tablespoons olive oil
- 4 cloves garlic, minced
- 1 tablespoon fresh rosemary, chopped
- 1 tablespoon fresh thyme, chopped
- 1/4 teaspoon black pepper
- 4 carrots, peeled and cut into chunks
- 4 parsnips, peeled and cut into chunks
- 2 sweet potatoes, peeled and cut into chunks
- 1 large onion, cut into wedges

Instructions:

1. Preheat the oven to 375°F (190°C).
2. In a small bowl, mix 2 tablespoons of olive oil, garlic, rosemary, thyme, and black pepper.
3. Rub the herb mixture all over the chicken.
4. Toss the vegetables with the remaining 2 tablespoons of olive oil and place them in a roasting pan.
5. Place the chicken on top of the vegetables.
6. Roast for 1.5-2 hours, until the chicken reaches an internal temperature of 165°F (74°C) and the vegetables are tender.
7. Let the chicken rest for 10 minutes before carving.
8. Serve immediately.

Nutrition Info per Serving:

- Calories: 450
- Protein: 40g
- Carbohydrates: 20g
- Fat: 24g
- Fiber: 4g
- Sugar: 6g

Number of Servings:

- **6 servings**

Cooking Time:

- **2 hours**

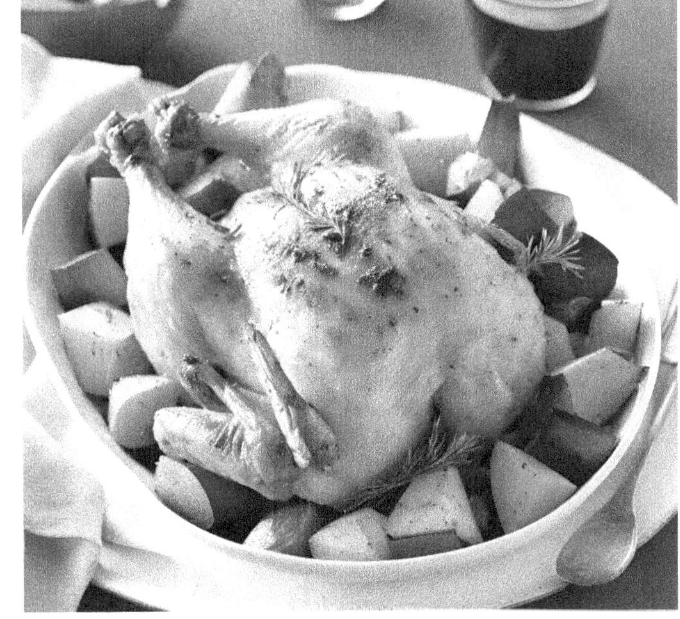

17. Chicken Salad with Greek Yogurt

Ingredients:

- 2 cups cooked chicken breast, diced
- 1/2 cup plain Greek yogurt
- 1 tablespoon Dijon mustard
- 1/2 cup celery, diced
- 1/4 cup red onion, finely chopped
- 1/4 cup dried cranberries
- 1/4 cup chopped walnuts
- 1/4 teaspoon black pepper
- 1 tablespoon fresh parsley, chopped (optional)

Instructions:

1. In a large bowl, combine the Greek yogurt, Dijon mustard, and black pepper.
2. Add the diced chicken, celery, red onion, dried cranberries, and walnuts. Mix until well combined.
3. Garnish with fresh parsley if desired.
4. Serve immediately or refrigerate until ready to serve.

Nutrition Info per Serving:

- Calories: 300
- Protein: 30g
- Carbohydrates: 12g
- Fat: 15g
- Fiber: 3g
- Sugar: 7g

Number of Servings:

- 4 servings

Cooking Time:

- 10 minutes (plus any time needed to cook the chicken)

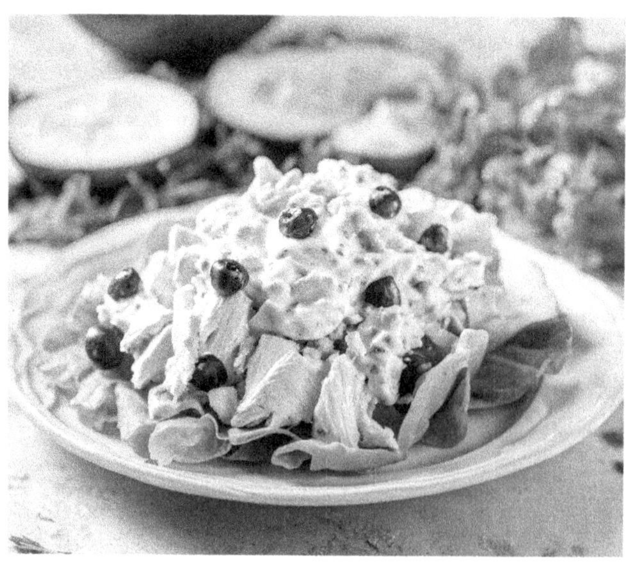

18. Turkey and Spinach Meatloaf

Ingredients:

- 1 pound ground turkey
- 1/2 cup cooked quinoa
- 1 egg, beaten
- 1/2 cup chopped spinach
- 1/2 cup diced onion
- 2 cloves garlic, minced
- 1 tablespoon Worcestershire sauce
- 1/4 teaspoon black pepper
- 1/2 cup tomato sauce (for topping)

Instructions:

1. Preheat the oven to 375°F (190°C) and grease a loaf pan.
2. In a large bowl, combine the ground turkey, cooked quinoa, beaten egg, spinach, onion, garlic, Worcestershire sauce, and black pepper. Mix until well combined.
3. Transfer the mixture to the prepared loaf pan and shape into a loaf.
4. Spread the tomato sauce evenly over the top.
5. Bake for 45-50 minutes, until the internal temperature reaches 165°F (74°C).
6. Let the meatloaf rest for 10 minutes before slicing.
7. Serve immediately.

Nutrition Info per Serving:

- Calories: 250
- Protein: 28g
- Carbohydrates: 12g
- Fat: 10g
- Fiber: 2g
- Sugar: 4g

Number of Servings:

- **4 servings**

Cooking Time:

- **50 minutes**

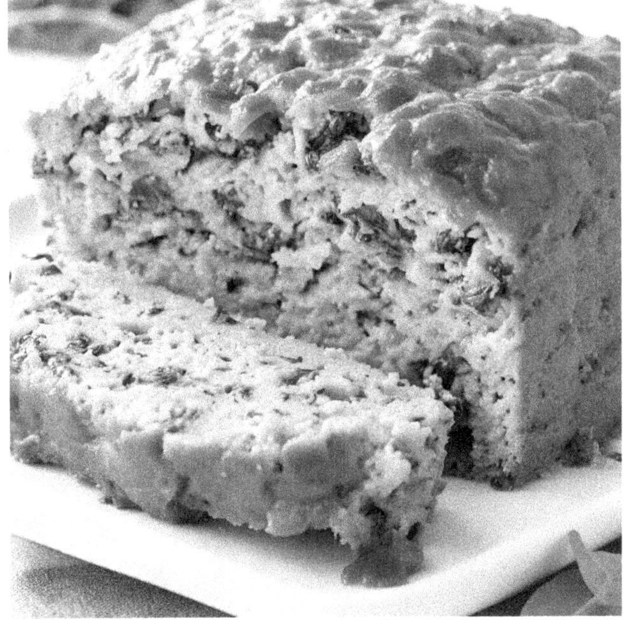

19. Cajun Chicken Skillet

Ingredients:

- 1 pound boneless, skinless chicken breasts, cut into strips
- 2 tablespoons olive oil
- 1 tablespoon Cajun seasoning
- 1 red bell pepper, sliced
- 1 green bell pepper, sliced
- 1 yellow bell pepper, sliced
- 1 onion, sliced
- 2 cloves garlic, minced
- 1/4 teaspoon black pepper
- 1/2 cup low-sodium chicken broth
- Fresh parsley for garnish (optional)

Instructions:

1. In a large bowl, toss the chicken strips with Cajun seasoning and black pepper.
2. Heat the olive oil in a large skillet over medium heat. Add the chicken and cook for 5-7 minutes until browned and cooked through. Remove from the skillet and set aside.
3. In the same skillet, add the bell peppers, onion, and garlic. Cook for 5-7 minutes until the vegetables are tender.
4. Return the chicken to the skillet and add the chicken broth. Cook for an additional 2-3 minutes until heated through.
5. Garnish with fresh parsley if desired.
6. Serve immediately.

Nutrition Info per Serving:

- Calories: 300
- Protein: 30g
- Carbohydrates: 10g
- Fat: 15g
- Fiber: 3g
- Sugar: 4g

Number of Servings:

- **4 servings**

Cooking Time:

- **20 minutes**

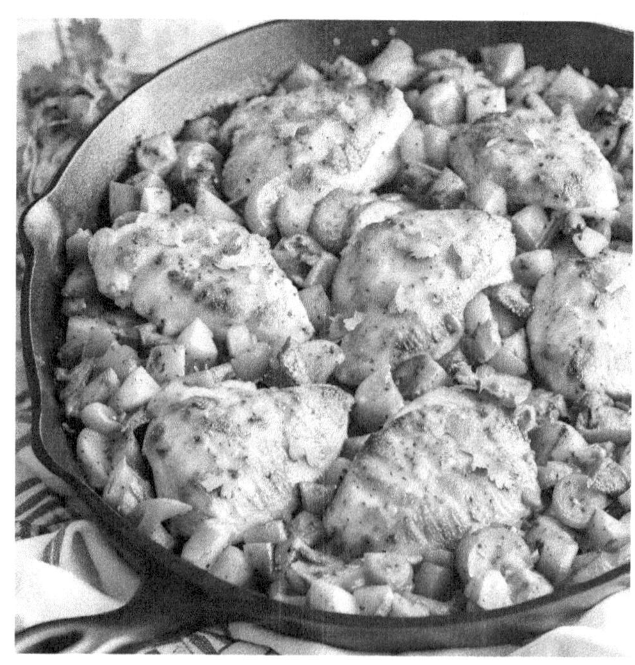

20. Pesto Chicken Bake

Ingredients:

- 4 boneless, skinless chicken breasts
- 1/2 cup pesto sauce
- 1/2 cup shredded mozzarella cheese
- 1/4 cup grated Parmesan cheese
- 1 cup cherry tomatoes, halved
- 2 tablespoons olive oil
- 1/4 teaspoon black pepper

Instructions:

1. Preheat the oven to 375°F (190°C).
2. Rub the chicken breasts with olive oil and black pepper. Place them in a baking dish.
3. Spread pesto sauce evenly over each chicken breast.
4. Sprinkle mozzarella and Parmesan cheese on top.
5. Scatter cherry tomatoes around the chicken in the baking dish.
6. Bake for 25-30 minutes, until the chicken is cooked through and the cheese is bubbly and golden.
7. Serve immediately.

Nutrition Info per Serving:

- Calories: 350
- Protein: 35g
- Carbohydrates: 5g
- Fat: 20g
- Fiber: 1g
- Sugar: 3g

Number of Servings:

- **4 servings**

Cooking Time:

- **30 minutes**

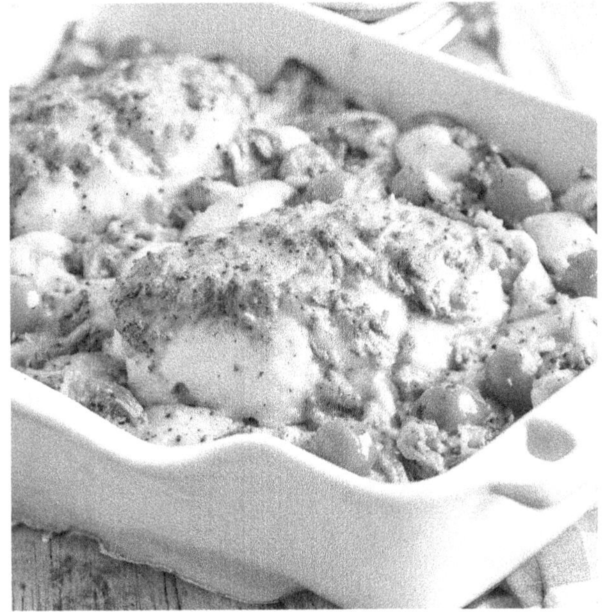

21. Chicken and Spinach Quiche

Ingredients:

- 1 pre-made whole wheat pie crust
- 1 cup cooked chicken breast, diced
- 1 cup fresh spinach, chopped
- 1/2 cup shredded Swiss cheese
- 1/2 cup milk
- 1/2 cup plain Greek yogurt
- 4 large eggs
- 1/4 teaspoon black pepper
- 1/4 teaspoon garlic powder

Instructions:

1. Preheat the oven to 350°F (175°C).
2. Place the pie crust in a 9-inch pie dish.
3. In a large bowl, whisk together the milk, Greek yogurt, eggs, black pepper, and garlic powder.
4. Spread the diced chicken and chopped spinach evenly over the pie crust.
5. Pour the egg mixture over the chicken and spinach.
6. Sprinkle the shredded Swiss cheese on top.
7. Bake for 35-40 minutes, until the quiche is set and golden brown.
8. Allow to cool for 5 minutes before slicing.
9. Serve immediately.

Nutrition Info per Serving:

- Calories: 300
- Protein: 20g
- Carbohydrates: 20g
- Fat: 15g
- Fiber: 2g
- Sugar: 4g

Number of Servings:

- **6 servings**

Cooking Time:

- **40 minutes**

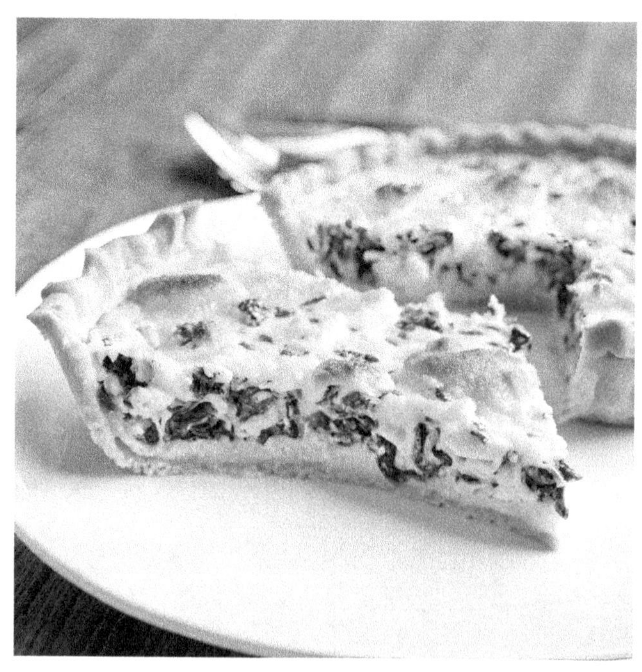

22. Balsamic Glazed Chicken

Ingredients:

- 4 boneless, skinless chicken breasts
- 2 tablespoons olive oil
- 1/4 cup balsamic vinegar
- 2 tablespoons honey
- 2 cloves garlic, minced
- 1/4 teaspoon black pepper

Instructions:

1. Heat the olive oil in a large skillet over medium heat.
2. Add the chicken breasts and cook for 5-7 minutes per side, until golden brown and cooked through.
3. Remove the chicken from the skillet and set aside.
4. In the same skillet, add the balsamic vinegar, honey, minced garlic, and black pepper. Cook for 2-3 minutes, until the sauce thickens slightly.
5. Return the chicken to the skillet and coat with the balsamic glaze.
6. Serve immediately.

Nutrition Info per Serving:

- Calories: 300
- Protein: 30g
- Carbohydrates: 12g
- Fat: 12g
- Fiber: 0g
- Sugar: 10g

Number of Servings:

- **4 servings**

Cooking Time:

- **20 minutes**

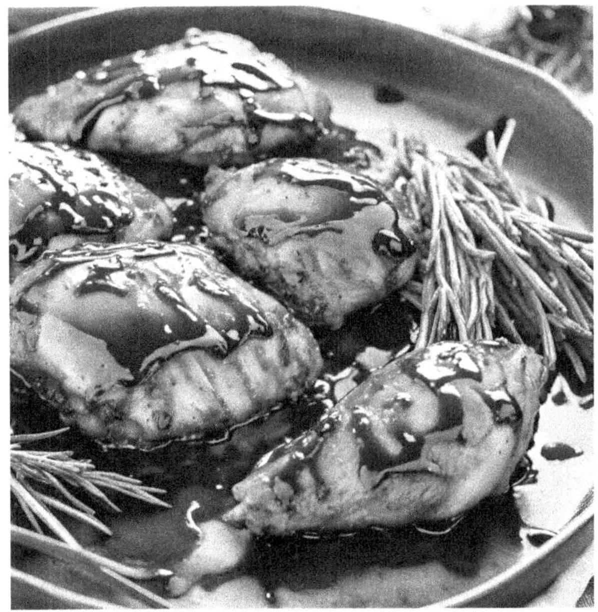

23. Chicken Noodle Soup

Ingredients:

- 1 pound boneless, skinless chicken breasts, diced
- 8 cups low-sodium chicken broth
- 2 carrots, sliced
- 2 celery stalks, sliced
- 1 onion, diced
- 2 cloves garlic, minced
- 1 teaspoon dried thyme
- 1/4 teaspoon black pepper
- 2 cups whole wheat egg noodles
- 2 tablespoons olive oil
- Fresh parsley for garnish (optional)

Instructions:

1. Heat olive oil in a large pot over medium heat. Add the onion, garlic, carrots, and celery. Cook until the vegetables are softened, about 5 minutes.
2. Add the diced chicken, chicken broth, thyme, and black pepper. Bring to a boil.
3. Reduce heat and simmer for 20 minutes, until the chicken is cooked through.
4. Add the whole wheat egg noodles and cook for an additional 10 minutes, until the noodles are tender.
5. Garnish with fresh parsley if desired.
6. Serve immediately.

Nutrition Info per Serving:

- Calories: 250
- Protein: 25g
- Carbohydrates: 25g
- Fat: 8g
- Fiber: 3g
- Sugar: 4g

Number of Servings:

- **6 servings**

Cooking Time:

- **35 minutes**

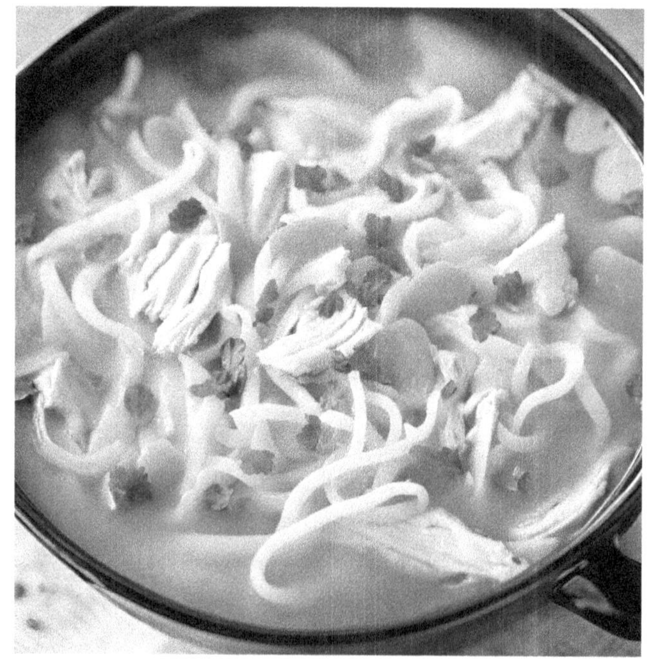

24. Dijon Mustard Chicken

Ingredients:

- 4 boneless, skinless chicken breasts
- 2 tablespoons olive oil
- 1/4 cup Dijon mustard
- 2 tablespoons honey
- 1 tablespoon lemon juice
- 2 cloves garlic, minced
- 1/4 teaspoon black pepper

Instructions:

1. Preheat the oven to 375°F (190°C).
2. In a small bowl, mix the Dijon mustard, honey, lemon juice, garlic, and black pepper.
3. Rub the chicken breasts with olive oil and place them in a baking dish.
4. Spread the mustard mixture evenly over the chicken breasts.
5. Bake for 25-30 minutes, until the chicken is cooked through and juices run clear.
6. Serve immediately.

Nutrition Info per Serving:

- Calories: 280
- Protein: 30g
- Carbohydrates: 10g
- Fat: 12g
- Fiber: 0g
- Sugar: 8g

Number of Servings:

- **4 servings**

Cooking Time:

- **30 minutes**

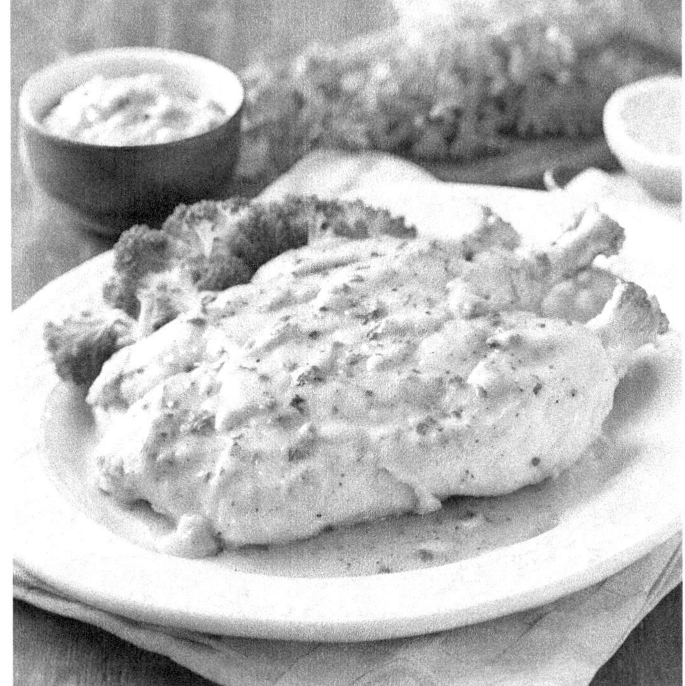

25. Chicken Vegetable Stir-Fry

Ingredients:

- 1 pound boneless, skinless chicken breasts, thinly sliced
- 2 tablespoons olive oil
- 1 red bell pepper, sliced
- 1 yellow bell pepper, sliced
- 1 green bell pepper, sliced
- 1 large onion, sliced
- 2 cloves garlic, minced
- 1/4 cup low-sodium soy sauce
- 1 tablespoon rice vinegar
- 1 tablespoon honey
- 1 teaspoon grated fresh ginger
- 1/4 teaspoon black pepper
- 2 cups cooked brown rice (for serving)

Instructions:

1. Heat 1 tablespoon of olive oil in a large skillet or wok over medium-high heat. Add the chicken and cook until browned and cooked through, about 5-7 minutes. Remove from the skillet and set aside.
2. Add the remaining 1 tablespoon of olive oil to the skillet. Add the bell peppers, onion, and garlic. Cook until the vegetables are tender, about 5-7 minutes.
3. In a small bowl, mix the soy sauce, rice vinegar, honey, grated ginger, and black pepper.
4. Return the chicken to the skillet and pour the sauce over the top. Cook for an additional 2-3 minutes, until everything is heated through.
5. Serve the stir-fry over cooked brown rice.
6. Serve immediately.

Nutrition Info per Serving:

- Calories: 350
- Protein: 30g
- Carbohydrates: 35g
- Fat: 10g
- Fiber: 4g
- Sugar: 10g

Number of Servings:

- **4 servings**

Cooking Time:

- **20 minutes**

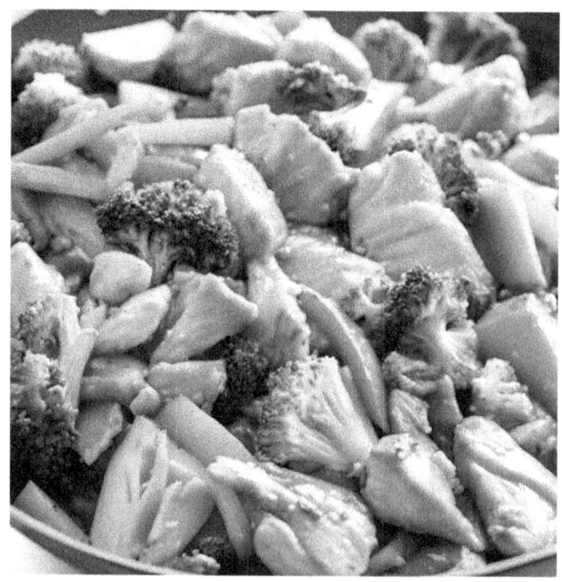

26. Baked Turkey Meatballs

Ingredients:

- 1 pound ground turkey
- 1/2 cup whole wheat breadcrumbs
- 1 egg, beaten
- 1/4 cup grated Parmesan cheese (optional)
- 2 cloves garlic, minced
- 1 tablespoon fresh parsley, chopped
- 1/4 teaspoon black pepper
- 1 tablespoon olive oil
- 1/2 cup marinara sauce (for serving)

Instructions:

1. Preheat the oven to 375°F (190°C) and line a baking sheet with parchment paper.
2. In a large bowl, combine the ground turkey, breadcrumbs, beaten egg, Parmesan cheese (if using), garlic, parsley, and black pepper. Mix until well combined.
3. Form the mixture into 1-inch meatballs and place them on the prepared baking sheet.
4. Brush the meatballs with olive oil.
5. Bake for 20-25 minutes, until the meatballs are cooked through and golden brown.
6. Serve with marinara sauce.
7. Serve immediately.

Nutrition Info per Serving:

- Calories: 220
- Protein: 25g
- Carbohydrates: 10g
- Fat: 10g
- Fiber: 1g
- Sugar: 2g

Number of Servings:

- **4 servings**

Cooking Time:

- **25 minutes**

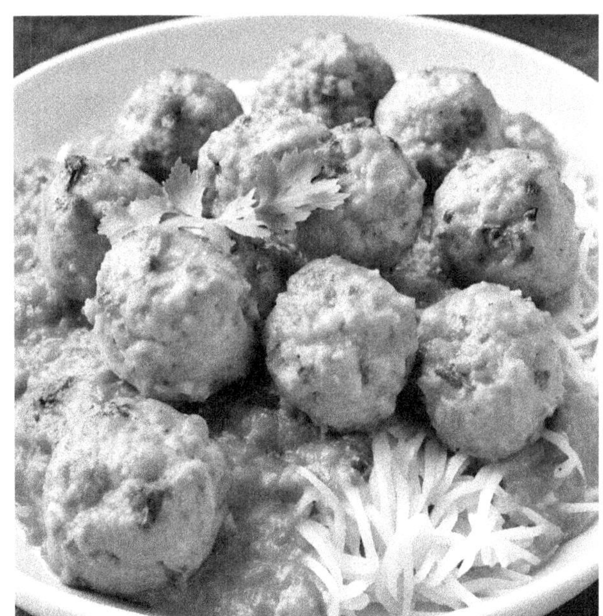

Soup & Stew Recipes

1. Tom Yum Goong

Ingredients:
- 1 pound large shrimp, peeled and deveined
- 4 cups low-sodium chicken broth
- 1 cup water
- 3 stalks lemongrass, cut into 2-inch pieces and smashed
- 3 kaffir lime leaves, torn into pieces
- 1-inch piece galangal, sliced
- 3 cloves garlic, minced
- 1 cup mushrooms, sliced
- 2-3 Thai red chilies, sliced
- 3 tablespoons fish sauce
- 2 tablespoons lime juice
- 1 tablespoon Thai chili paste (Nam Prik Pao)
- 1/2 cup cherry tomatoes, halved
- 1/4 cup fresh cilantro, chopped

Instructions:
1. In a large pot, bring the chicken broth and water to a boil.
2. Add the lemongrass, kaffir lime leaves, galangal, and garlic. Simmer for 10 minutes.
3. Add the mushrooms and Thai chilies. Cook for another 5 minutes.
4. Stir in the fish sauce, lime juice, and Thai chili paste.
5. Add the shrimp and cherry tomatoes. Cook for 3-4 minutes until the shrimp are pink and cooked through.
6. Remove from heat and garnish with fresh cilantro.
7. Serve immediately.

Nutrition Info per Serving:
- Calories: 180
- Protein: 18g
- Carbohydrates: 10g
- Fat: 7g
- Fiber: 2g
- Sugar: 3g

Number of Servings:
- 4 servings

Cooking Time:
- 20 minutes

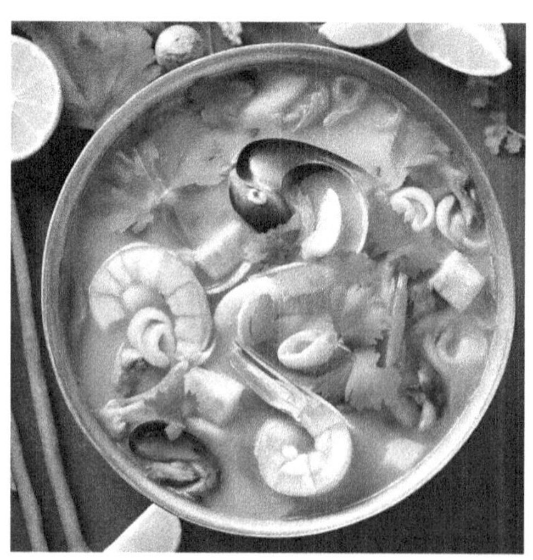

2. Corned Beef and Cabbage Soup

Ingredients:

- 1 pound corned beef, cooked and diced
- 6 cups low-sodium beef broth
- 1 cup water
- 1 large onion, diced
- 3 cloves garlic, minced
- 4 carrots, sliced
- 4 celery stalks, sliced
- 2 cups cabbage, chopped
- 1 teaspoon dried thyme
- 1/4 teaspoon black pepper
- 2 cups potatoes, peeled and diced

Instructions:

1. In a large pot, heat a tablespoon of olive oil over medium heat. Add the onion and garlic, and cook until softened, about 5 minutes.
2. Add the carrots, celery, and potatoes. Cook for another 5 minutes.
3. Pour in the beef broth and water. Stir in the thyme and black pepper. Bring to a boil.
4. Reduce heat and simmer for 20 minutes until the vegetables are tender.
5. Add the corned beef and cabbage. Cook for an additional 10 minutes.
6. Serve immediately.

Nutrition Info per Serving:

- Calories: 250
- Protein: 18g
- Carbohydrates: 25g
- Fat: 8g
- Fiber: 5g
- Sugar: 5g

Number of Servings:

- **6 servings**

Cooking Time:

- **35 minutes**

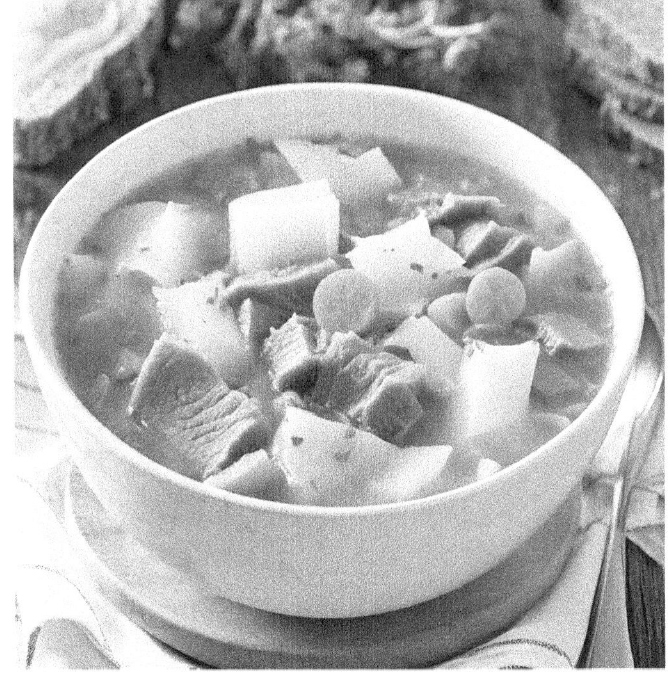

3. Black Bean Soup

Ingredients:

- 2 cups dried black beans, soaked overnight
- 6 cups low-sodium vegetable broth
- 1 large onion, diced
- 3 cloves garlic, minced
- 2 carrots, diced
- 2 celery stalks, diced
- 1 red bell pepper, diced
- 1 teaspoon cumin
- 1 teaspoon dried oregano
- 1/4 teaspoon black pepper
- 1 tablespoon olive oil
- 2 tablespoons lime juice
- Fresh cilantro for garnish (optional)

Instructions:

1. Heat olive oil in a large pot over medium heat. Add the onion and garlic, and cook until softened, about 5 minutes.
2. Add the carrots, celery, and red bell pepper. Cook for another 5 minutes.
3. Stir in the cumin, oregano, and black pepper.
4. Add the soaked black beans and vegetable broth. Bring to a boil.
5. Reduce heat and simmer for 1.5-2 hours until the beans are tender.
6. Use an immersion blender to puree part of the soup to your desired consistency.
7. Stir in the lime juice.
8. Serve immediately, garnished with fresh cilantro if desired.

Nutrition Info per Serving:

- Calories: 220
- Protein: 12g
- Carbohydrates: 40g
- Fat: 4g
- Fiber: 12g
- Sugar: 5g

Number of Servings:

- **6 servings**

Cooking Time:

- **2 hours**

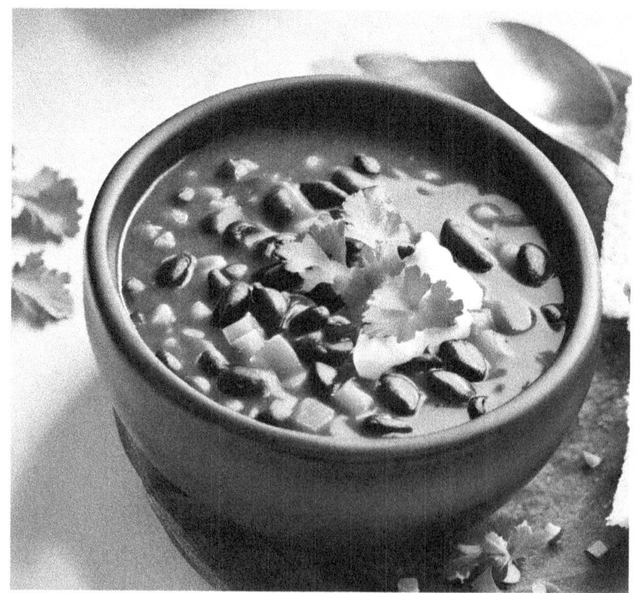

4. Chicken Gumbo
Ingredients:
- 1 pound boneless, skinless chicken thighs, diced
- 1/2 pound andouille sausage, sliced
- 6 cups low-sodium chicken broth
- 1 large onion, diced
- 1 green bell pepper, diced
- 2 celery stalks, diced
- 3 cloves garlic, minced
- 1 cup okra, sliced
- 1 can (14.5 ounces) diced tomatoes
- 1/2 cup flour
- 1/2 cup vegetable oil
- 1 teaspoon dried thyme
- 1 teaspoon paprika
- 1/4 teaspoon black pepper
- 1/4 teaspoon cayenne pepper (optional)
- 1 bay leaf
- 1 cup cooked brown rice (for serving)

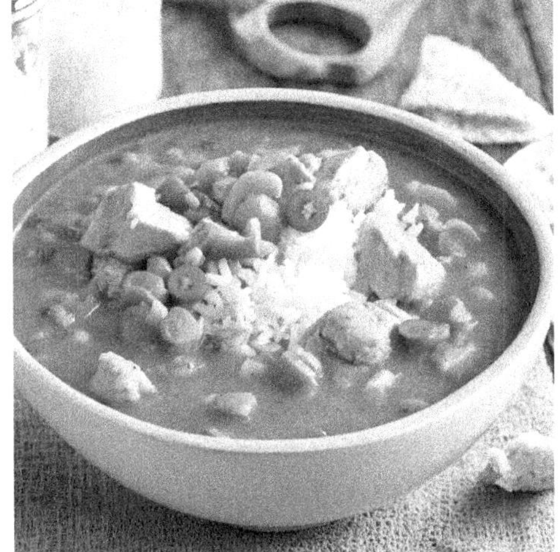

Instructions:
1. In a large pot, heat the vegetable oil over medium heat. Gradually whisk in the flour to make a roux. Cook, stirring constantly, until the roux is a deep brown color, about 15-20 minutes.
2. Add the onion, bell pepper, celery, and garlic to the roux. Cook for 5 minutes until softened.
3. Stir in the diced chicken and andouille sausage. Cook for another 5 minutes.
4. Add the okra, diced tomatoes, chicken broth, thyme, paprika, black pepper, cayenne pepper (if using), and bay leaf. Bring to a boil.
5. Reduce heat and simmer for 45 minutes.
6. Remove the bay leaf before serving.
7. Serve the gumbo over cooked brown rice.
8. Serve immediately.

Nutrition Info per Serving:
- Calories: 400
- Protein: 25g
- Carbohydrates: 35g
- Fat: 18g
- Fiber: 5g
- Sugar: 4g

Number of Servings:
- **6 servings**

Cooking Time:
- **1 hour 15 minutes**

5. Manhattan Clam Chowder

Ingredients:

- 2 cups clams, chopped
- 6 cups low-sodium clam juice
- 1 large onion, diced
- 3 cloves garlic, minced
- 2 carrots, diced
- 2 celery stalks, diced
- 1 large potato, diced
- 1 can (14.5 ounces) diced tomatoes
- 1 tablespoon tomato paste
- 1 teaspoon dried thyme
- 1/4 teaspoon black pepper
- 2 tablespoons olive oil
- 1 bay leaf

Instructions:

1. Heat olive oil in a large pot over medium heat. Add the onion and garlic, and cook until softened, about 5 minutes.
2. Add the carrots, celery, and potato. Cook for another 5 minutes.
3. Stir in the diced tomatoes, tomato paste, thyme, black pepper, and bay leaf.
4. Pour in the clam juice and bring to a boil.
5. Reduce heat and simmer for 20 minutes until the vegetables are tender.
6. Add the chopped clams and cook for an additional 5 minutes.
7. Remove the bay leaf before serving.
8. Serve immediately.

Nutrition Info per Serving:

- Calories: 250
- Protein: 20g
- Carbohydrates: 25g
- Fat: 8g
- Fiber: 4g
- Sugar: 6g

Number of Servings:

- **6 servings**

Cooking Time:

- **35 minutes**

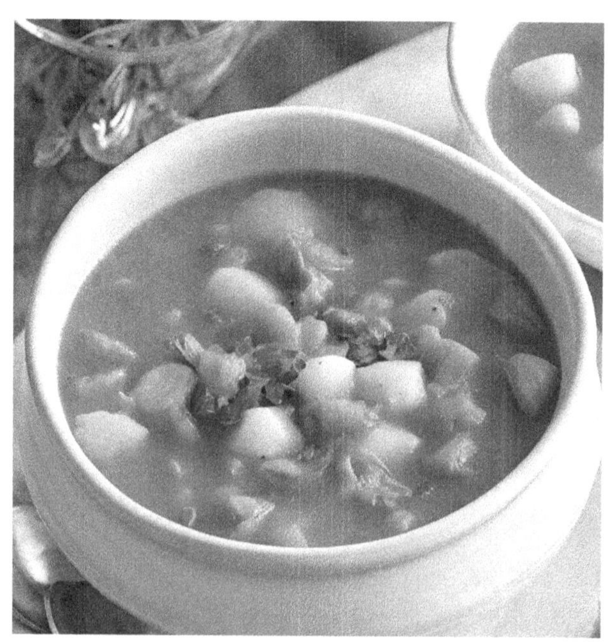

6. Cream of Mushroom Soup

Ingredients:

- 1 pound mushrooms, sliced
- 1 large onion, diced
- 3 cloves garlic, minced
- 4 cups low-sodium vegetable broth
- 1 cup milk or dairy-free milk
- 2 tablespoons flour
- 2 tablespoons olive oil
- 1 teaspoon dried thyme
- 1/4 teaspoon black pepper
- 1/4 cup fresh parsley, chopped (optional)

Instructions:

1. Heat olive oil in a large pot over medium heat. Add the onion and garlic, and cook until softened, about 5 minutes.
2. Add the sliced mushrooms and cook until they release their juices, about 10 minutes.
3. Stir in the flour and cook for another 2 minutes.
4. Gradually add the vegetable broth, stirring constantly to prevent lumps.
5. Stir in the thyme and black pepper. Bring to a boil.
6. Reduce heat and simmer for 15 minutes.
7. Use an immersion blender to puree the soup to your desired consistency.
8. Stir in the milk and cook for another 5 minutes until heated through.
9. Garnish with fresh parsley if desired.
10. Serve immediately.

Nutrition Info per Serving:

- Calories: 180
- Protein: 6g
- Carbohydrates: 18g
- Fat: 10g
- Fiber: 2g
- Sugar: 5g

Number of Servings:

- **4 servings**

Cooking Time:

- **35 minutes**

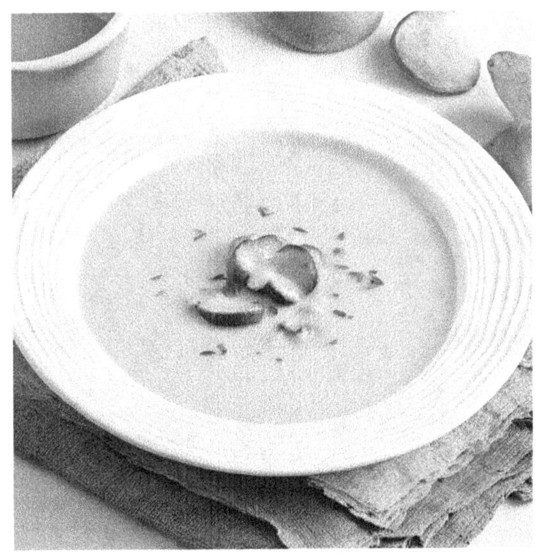

7. Hot and Sour Soup

Ingredients:

- 1/2 pound tofu, cut into small cubes
- 6 cups low-sodium vegetable broth
- 1 cup mushrooms, sliced
- 1 cup bamboo shoots, julienned
- 1 carrot, julienned
- 1/4 cup rice vinegar
- 3 tablespoons low-sodium soy sauce
- 2 tablespoons cornstarch mixed with 2 tablespoons water
- 1 tablespoon chili paste
- 1 tablespoon grated fresh ginger
- 2 cloves garlic, minced
- 2 eggs, beaten
- 1/4 teaspoon black pepper
- 2 green onions, sliced (optional for garnish)

Instructions:

1. In a large pot, bring the vegetable broth to a boil.
2. Add the mushrooms, bamboo shoots, carrot, rice vinegar, soy sauce, chili paste, ginger, and garlic. Simmer for 10 minutes.
3. Stir in the cornstarch mixture and cook for 2-3 minutes until the soup thickens slightly.
4. Add the tofu and cook for another 2 minutes.
5. Slowly drizzle in the beaten eggs while stirring the soup to create egg ribbons.
6. Garnish with sliced green onions if desired.
7. Serve immediately.

Nutrition Info per Serving:

- Calories: 150
- Protein: 8g
- Carbohydrates: 12g
- Fat: 8g
- Fiber: 2g
- Sugar: 3g

Number of Servings:

- **4 servings**

Cooking Time:

- **20 minutes**

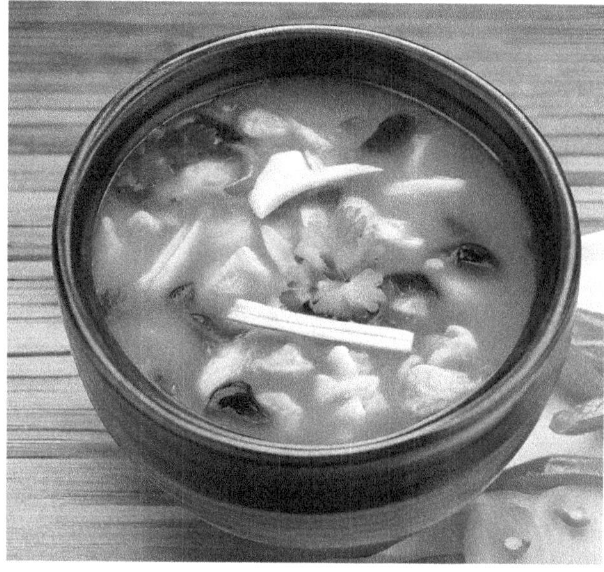

10-WEEK MEAL PLAN

Week 1

Day 1:
- Breakfast: Scrambled Eggs with Spinach
- Lunch: Black Bean Soup
- Dinner: Baked Cod with Lemon and Capers
- Snack: Greek Yogurt with Fresh Berries

Day 2:
- Breakfast: Banana Pancakes
- Lunch: Chicken Salad with Greek Yogurt
- Dinner: Chicken Provençal
- Snack: Apple Slices with Almond Butter

Day 3:
- Breakfast: Smoothie Bowl
- Lunch: Lentil and Vegetable Stew
- Dinner: Balsamic Glazed Chicken
- Snack: Carrot Sticks with Hummus

Day 4:
- Breakfast: Oatmeal with Fresh Berries
- Lunch: Mediterranean Turkey Patties
- Dinner: Sea Bass with Mango Salsa
- Snack: Mixed Nuts

Day 5:
- Breakfast: Apple Cinnamon Porridge
- Lunch: Chicken Noodle Soup
- Dinner: Grilled Salmon with Dill Sauce
- Snack: Cottage Cheese with Pineapple

Day 6:
- Breakfast: Egg and Vegetable Muffins
- Lunch: Turkey Sloppy Joes
- Dinner: Shrimp Stir-Fry
- Snack: Celery Sticks with Peanut Butter

Day 7:
- Breakfast: Sweet Potato Hash
- Lunch: Chicken Gumbo
- Dinner: Tilapia with Tomato Basil Sauce
- Snack: Fresh Fruit Salad

Week 2

Day 8:

- Breakfast: Quinoa and Berry Breakfast Bowl
- Lunch: Corned Beef and Cabbage Soup
- Dinner: Smoked Paprika Chicken
- Snack: Trail Mix

Day 9:

- Breakfast: Turkey and Spinach Omelette
- Lunch: Cucumber Gazpacho
- Dinner: Roasted Cauliflower Steaks
- Snack: Yogurt with Honey and Walnuts

Day 10:

- Breakfast: Almond Butter and Banana Sandwich
- Lunch: Chicken Fajitas
- Dinner: Baked Trout with Almonds
- Snack: Bell Pepper Slices with Guacamole

Day 11:

- Breakfast: Chia Pudding
- Lunch: Chicken Minestrone Soup
- Dinner: Roasted Brussels Sprouts with Garlic and Chicken
- Snack: Roasted Chickpeas

Day 12:

- Breakfast: Buckwheat Pancakes
- Lunch: Eggplant Parmesan
- Dinner: Fish Tacos with Cabbage Slaw
- Snack: Grapes and Cheese Cubes

Day 13:

- Breakfast: Kale and Mushroom Sauté
- Lunch: Chicken and Pea Risotto
- Dinner: Pan-Fried Mackerel with Lemon
- Snack: Rice Cakes with Avocado

Day 14:

- Breakfast: Baked Avocado Eggs
- Lunch: Chicken Vegetable Stir-Fry
- Dinner: Grilled Mahi Mahi with Pineapple Salsa
- Snack: Smoothie with Spinach, Banana, and Almond Milk

Week 3

Day 15:

- Breakfast: Millet Porridge
- Lunch: Vegetable Stir-Fry
- Dinner: Shrimp and Asparagus Risotto
- Snack: Apple with Sunflower Seed Butter

Day 16:

- Breakfast: Zucchini Bread
- Lunch: Turkey and Quinoa Stuffed Zucchini
- Dinner: Chicken Paillard
- Snack: Cucumber Slices with Cream Cheese

Day 17:

- Breakfast: Tofu Scramble
- Lunch: Manhattan Clam Chowder
- Dinner: Halibut with Herb Butter
- Snack: Edamame

Day 18:

- Breakfast: Peanut Butter and Jelly Oatmeal
- Lunch: Lentil and Vegetable Stew
- Dinner: Monkfish Stew
- Snack: Almonds and Raisins

Day 19:

- Breakfast: Broccoli and Cheese Frittata
- Lunch: Green Beans Almondine
- Dinner: Baked Lemon Sole with Capers
- Snack: Kale Chips

Day 20:

- Breakfast: Pear and Walnut Oatmeal
- Lunch: Chicken Provençal
- Dinner: Seared Tuna with Sesame Seeds
- Snack: Cherry Tomatoes with Feta

Day 21:

- Breakfast: Vegetable and Quinoa Breakfast Bowl
- Lunch: Spaghetti Squash Primavera
- Dinner: Fish Soup with Tomatoes
- Snack: Orange Slices

Week 4

Day 22:

- Breakfast: Almond Flour Blueberry Muffins
- Lunch: Butternut Squash Risotto
- Dinner: Seared Scallops with Pea Puree
- Snack: Pear with Ricotta Cheese

Day 23:

- Breakfast: Egg White and Avocado Wrap
- Lunch: Hot and Sour Soup
- Dinner: Pesto Chicken Bake
- Snack: Strawberries with Balsamic Vinegar

Day 24:
- Breakfast: Sweet Corn and Zucchini Pancakes
- Lunch: Turkey Sloppy Joes
- Dinner: Fish Curry with Coconut Milk
- Snack: Mixed Seeds

Day 25:
- Breakfast: Raspberry Chia Jam on Toast
- Lunch: Curried Cauliflower Soup
- Dinner: Perch with Creamy Dill Sauce
- Snack: Apple Slices with Almond Butter

Day 26:
- Breakfast: Soy Yogurt with Compote
- Lunch: Chicken and Spinach Quiche
- Dinner: Snapper Veracruz
- Snack: Greek Yogurt with Granola

Day 27:
- Breakfast: Turkey and Spinach Omelette
- Lunch: Vegetable and Quinoa Breakfast Bowl
- Dinner: Pan-Seared Duck Breast
- Snack: Cottage Cheese with Pineapple

Day 28:
- Breakfast: Kale and Mushroom Sauté
- Lunch: Roasted Turnips with Rosemary
- Dinner: Chicken Gumbo
- Snack: Fresh Fruit Salad

Week 5

Day 29:
- Breakfast: Almond Butter and Banana Sandwich
- Lunch: Roasted Brussels Sprouts with Garlic
- Dinner: Turkey and Spinach Meatloaf
- Snack: Yogurt with Honey and Walnuts

Day 30:
- Breakfast: Zucchini Bread
- Lunch: Lentil and Vegetable Stew
- Dinner: Balsamic Glazed Chicken
- Snack: Bell Pepper Slices with Guacamole

Day 31:
- Breakfast: Tofu Scramble
- Lunch: Manhattan Clam Chowder
- Dinner: Halibut with Herb Butter
- Snack: Roasted Chickpeas

Day 32:
- Breakfast: Peanut Butter and Jelly Oatmeal
- Lunch: Turkey and Quinoa Stuffed Zucchini
- Dinner: Chicken Paillard
- Snack: Edamame

Day 33:
- Breakfast: Broccoli and Cheese Frittata
- Lunch: Spaghetti Squash Primavera
- Dinner: Monkfish Stew
- Snack: Kale Chips

Day 34:
- Breakfast: Pear and Walnut Oatmeal
- Lunch: Green Beans Almondine
- Dinner: Baked Lemon Sole with Capers
- Snack: Almonds and Raisins

Day 35:
- Breakfast: Vegetable and Quinoa Breakfast Bowl
- Lunch: Butternut Squash Risotto
- Dinner: Fish Soup with Tomatoes
- Snack: Cherry Tomatoes with Feta

Week 6

Day 36:
- Breakfast: Smoothie with Spinach, Banana, and Almond Milk
- Lunch: Chicken and Vegetable Stir-Fry
- Dinner: Grilled Swordfish with Herb Salad
- Snack: Apple Slices with Peanut Butter

Day 37:
- Breakfast: Greek Yogurt with Fresh Berries and Honey
- Lunch: Roasted Cauliflower Steaks
- Dinner: Shrimp and Asparagus Risotto
- Snack: Carrot Sticks with Hummus

Day 38:
- Breakfast: Egg and Vegetable Muffins
- Lunch: Chicken Salad with Greek Yogurt
- Dinner: Sea Bass with Mango Salsa
- Snack: Mixed Nuts

Day 39:

- Breakfast: Sweet Potato Hash
- Lunch: Curried Cauliflower Soup
- Dinner: Pan-Fried Mackerel with Lemon
- Snack: Rice Cakes with Avocado

Day 40:

- Breakfast: Tofu Scramble
- Lunch: Spaghetti Squash Primavera
- Dinner: Seared Tuna with Sesame Seeds
- Snack: Bell Pepper Slices with Hummus

Day 41:

- Breakfast: Chia Pudding with Fresh Fruit
- Lunch: Chicken and Spinach Quiche
- Dinner: Grilled Mahi Mahi with Pineapple Salsa
- Snack: Trail Mix

Day 42:

- Breakfast: Kale and Mushroom Sauté
- Lunch: Vegetable and Quinoa Breakfast Bowl
- Dinner: Baked Lemon Sole with Capers
- Snack: Cottage Cheese with Pineapple

Week 7

Day 43:

- Breakfast: Almond Butter and Banana Sandwich
- Lunch: Hot and Sour Soup
- Dinner: Chicken Paillard
- Snack: Celery Sticks with Peanut Butter

Day 44:

- Breakfast: Zucchini Bread
- Lunch: Manhattan Clam Chowder
- Dinner: Balsamic Glazed Chicken
- Snack: Roasted Chickpeas

Day 45:

- Breakfast: Peanut Butter and Jelly Oatmeal
- Lunch: Turkey and Quinoa Stuffed Zucchini
- Dinner: Monkfish Stew
- Snack: Edamame

Day 46:

- Breakfast: Broccoli and Cheese Frittata
- Lunch: Spaghetti Squash Primavera
- Dinner: Halibut with Herb Butter
- Snack: Kale Chips

Day 47:
- Breakfast: Pear and Walnut Oatmeal
- Lunch: Lentil and Vegetable Stew
- Dinner: Perch with Creamy Dill Sauce
- Snack: Greek Yogurt with Granola

Day 48:
- Breakfast: Vegetable and Quinoa Breakfast Bowl
- Lunch: Chicken Gumbo
- Dinner: Snapper Veracruz
- Snack: Mixed Seeds

Day 49:
- Breakfast: Almond Flour Blueberry Muffins
- Lunch: Roasted Brussels Sprouts with Garlic
- Dinner: Shrimp Stir-Fry
- Snack: Fresh Fruit Salad

Week 8

Day 50:
- Breakfast: Egg White and Avocado Wrap
- Lunch: Green Beans Almondine
- Dinner: Pan-Seared Duck Breast
- Snack: Apple Slices with Almond Butter

Day 51:
- Breakfast: Sweet Corn and Zucchini Pancakes
- Lunch: Butternut Squash Risotto
- Dinner: Baked Cod with Lemon and Capers
- Snack: Cottage Cheese with Fresh Pineapple

Day 52:
- Breakfast: Raspberry Chia Jam on Toast
- Lunch: Cucumber Gazpacho
- Dinner: Grilled Salmon with Dill Sauce
- Snack: Mixed Nuts

Day 53:
- Breakfast: Soy Yogurt with Compote
- Lunch: Chicken Salad with Greek Yogurt
- Dinner: Fish Curry with Coconut Milk
- Snack: Carrot Sticks with Hummus

Day 54:
- Breakfast: Quinoa and Berry Breakfast Bowl
- Lunch: Turkey Sloppy Joes
- Dinner: Pan-Fried Mackerel with Lemon
- Snack: Apple Slices with Peanut Butter

Day 55:
- Breakfast: Kale and Mushroom Sauté
- Lunch: Chicken and Pea Risotto
- Dinner: Seared Tuna with Sesame Seeds
- Snack: Rice Cakes with Avocado

Day 56:
- Breakfast: Smoothie with Spinach, Banana, and Almond Milk
- Lunch: Hot and Sour Soup
- Dinner: Baked Lemon Sole with Capers
- Snack: Bell Pepper Slices with Guacamole

Week 9

Day 57:
- Breakfast: Greek Yogurt with Fresh Berries and Honey
- Lunch: Chicken Minestrone Soup
- Dinner: Sea Bass with Mango Salsa
- Snack: Mixed Nuts

Day 58:
- Breakfast: Almond Butter and Banana Sandwich
- Lunch: Lentil and Vegetable Stew
- Dinner: Tilapia with Tomato Basil Sauce
- Snack: Carrot Sticks with Hummus

Day 59:
- Breakfast: Egg and Vegetable Muffins
- Lunch: Manhattan Clam Chowder
- Dinner: Chicken Provençal
- Snack: Apple Slices with Almond Butter

Day 60:
- Breakfast: Tofu Scramble
- Lunch: Green Beans Almondine
- Dinner: Monkfish Stew
- Snack: Roasted Chickpeas

Day 61:
- Breakfast: Peanut Butter and Jelly Oatmeal
- Lunch: Spaghetti Squash Primavera
- Dinner: Grilled Mahi Mahi with Pineapple Salsa
- Snack: Edamame

Day 62:
- Breakfast: Broccoli and Cheese Frittata
- Lunch: Chicken Salad with Greek Yogurt
- Dinner: Pan-Seared Duck Breast
- Snack: Kale Chips

Day 63:
- Breakfast: Pear and Walnut Oatmeal
- Lunch: Hot and Sour Soup
- Dinner: Halibut with Herb Butter
- Snack: Greek Yogurt with Granola

Week 10

Day 64:
- Breakfast: Vegetable and Quinoa Breakfast Bowl
- Lunch: Turkey Sloppy Joes
- Dinner: Snapper Veracruz
- Snack: Mixed Seeds

Day 65:
- Breakfast: Almond Flour Blueberry Muffins
- Lunch: Chicken Gumbo
- Dinner: Balsamic Glazed Chicken
- Snack: Fresh Fruit Salad

Day 66:
- Breakfast: Egg White and Avocado Wrap
- Lunch: Butternut Squash Risotto
- Dinner: Shrimp Stir-Fry
- Snack: Cottage Cheese with Pineapple

Day 67:
- Breakfast: Sweet Corn and Zucchini Pancakes
- Lunch: Roasted Brussels Sprouts with Garlic
- Dinner: Fish Curry with Coconut Milk
- Snack: Mixed Nuts

Day 68:
- Breakfast: Raspberry Chia Jam on Toast
- Lunch: Turkey and Quinoa Stuffed Zucchini
- Dinner: Baked Cod with Lemon and Capers
- Snack: Carrot Sticks with Hummus

Day 69:
- Breakfast: Soy Yogurt with Compote
- Lunch: Cucumber Gazpacho
- Dinner: Seared Tuna with Sesame Seeds
- Snack: Apple Slices with Almond Butter

Day 70:
- Breakfast: Quinoa and Berry Breakfast Bowl
- Lunch: Chicken and Pea Risotto
- Dinner: Grilled Swordfish with Herb Salad
- Snack: Bell Pepper Slices with Guacamole

Weekly Meal planner + Journal

	BREAKFAST	LUNCH	DINNER	SNACKS
MON				
TUE				
WED				
THU				
FRI				
SAT				
SUN				

What are your main goals for starting the brain cancer diet? (e.g., improving energy levels, managing side effects of treatment, enhancing overall health) What specific outcomes are you hoping to achieve by following this diet?

....

....

....

....

....

Weekly Meal planner + Journal

	BREAKFAST	LUNCH	DINNER	SNACKS
MON				
TUE				
WED				
THU				
FRI				
SAT				
SUN				

What do you know about the nutritional needs of brain cancer patients? Are there any particular nutrients you know are important for brain cancer patients? List them.

....

....

....

....

....

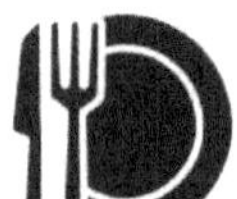

Weekly Meal planner + Journal

	BREAKFAST	LUNCH	DINNER	SNACKS
MON				
TUE				
WED				
THU				
FRI				
SAT				
SUN				

What challenges do you anticipate facing when starting the brain cancer diet? How do you plan to address these challenges?

Weekly Meal planner + Journal

	BREAKFAST	LUNCH	DINNER	SNACKS
MON				
TUE				
WED				
THU				
FRI				
SAT				
SUN				

What are your favorite foods and meals? Are there any foods or ingredients you dislike or have an aversion to?

Weekly Meal planner + Journal

	BREAKFAST	LUNCH	DINNER	SNACKS
MON				
TUE				
WED				
THU				
FRI				
SAT				
SUN				

How do you currently plan your meals? Do you use any specific tools or strategies? How do you think meal planning might change once you start following the brain cancer diet?

....

....

....

....

....

Weekly Meal planner + Journal

	BREAKFAST	LUNCH	DINNER	SNACKS
MON				
TUE				
WED				
THU				
FRI				
SAT				
SUN				

Describe your level of confidence in cooking. Are there any cooking techniques you are particularly good at or ones you want to learn? What kitchen equipment or tools do you find most helpful for preparing healthy meals?

Weekly Meal planner + Journal

	BREAKFAST	LUNCH	DINNER	SNACKS
MON				
TUE				
WED				
THU				
FRI				
SAT				
SUN				

Who in your life will support you in following this diet? How will they help you stay on track? Are there any support groups or resources you plan to utilize?

....

....

....

....

....

Weekly Meal planner + Journal

	BREAKFAST	LUNCH	DINNER	SNACKS
MON				
TUE				
WED				
THU				
FRI				
SAT				
SUN				

What symptoms related to brain cancer or its treatment do you currently experience? How do you think your diet might help manage these symptoms?

....

....

....

....

....

Weekly Meal planner + Journal

	BREAKFAST	LUNCH	DINNER	SNACKS
MON				
TUE				
WED				
THU				
FRI				
SAT				
SUN				

How will you reflect on your experiences with the brain cancer diet? Will you keep a journal or have regular check-ins with a healthcare provider? What will you do if you find that certain aspects of the diet are not working for you? How will you adjust your approach?

....

....

....

....

....

Scan the QR code below to get a surprise bonus